Calming Your Anxious Child

Calming Your Anxious Child

Words to Say and Things to Do

Kathleen Trainor, PsyD

JOHNS HOPKINS UNIVERSITY PRESS | Baltimore

Note to the reader: This book is not meant to substitute for medical care of children with anxiety, and treatment should not be based solely on its contents. Instead, treatment must be developed in a dialogue between the individual and his or her physician. This book has been written to help with that dialogue.

Drug dosage: The author and publisher have made reasonable efforts to determine that the selection of drugs discussed in this text conform to the practices of the general medical community. The medications described do not necessarily have specific approval by the U.S. Food and Drug Administration for use in the diseases for which they are recommended. In view of ongoing research, changes in governmental regulation, and the constant flow of information relating to drug therapy and drug reactions, the reader is urged to check the package insert of each drug for any change in indications and dosage and for warnings and precautions. This is particularly important when the recommended agent is a new and/or infrequently used drug.

© 2016 Kathleen Trainor
All rights reserved. Published 2016
Printed in the United States of America on acid-free paper
9 8 7 6 5 4 3 2 1

Johns Hopkins University Press
2715 North Charles Street
Baltimore, Maryland 21218-4363
www.press.jhu.edu

Library of Congress Cataloging-in-Publication Data

Trainor, Kathleen, 1955– author.
  Calming your anxious child : words to say and things to do / Kathleen Trainor.
Description: Baltimore : Johns Hopkins University Press, 2016. | Includes
    bibliographical references and index.
Identifiers: LCCN 2015034014| ISBN 9781421420097 (hardcover : alk. paper) |
    ISBN 9781421420103 (pbk. : alk. paper) | ISBN 9781421420110 (electronic) |
    ISBN 1421420090 (hardcover : alk. paper) | ISBN 1421420104 (pbk. : alk.
    paper) | ISBN 1421420112 (electronic)
Subjects: LCSH: Anxiety in children--Popular works. | Anxiety
    disorders--Treatment--Popular works. | Parent and child--Popular works.
Classification: LCC RJ506.A58 T73 2016 | DDC 618.92/8522--dc23 LC record available at
    http://lccn.loc.gov/2015034014

*Special discounts are available for bulk purchases of this book. For more information,
please contact Special Sales at 410-516-6936 or specialsales@press.jhu.edu.*

Johns Hopkins University Press uses environmentally friendly book materials, including recycled text paper that is composed of at least 30 percent post-consumer waste, whenever possible.

To all my patients, past and present,
who have been my greatest teachers.

To my children, Dagan, Brian,
and Kara, and my daughters-in-
law, Lori and Liza, and my beautiful
grandchildren, Dallan, Nevan,
and Braden.

My family has provided my inspiration
through their endless love and support.

Contents

Calming Your Anxious Child

Anxious about Anxiety

Responding to a Call for Help

Anxiety among children and adolescents is now considered an epidemic, and its prevalence continues to increase dramatically. After thirty-plus years of treating thousands of patients as a social worker and a child psychologist, I am amazed by the current pervasiveness of anxiety-related disorders such as obsessive compulsive disorder, separation anxiety, post-traumatic stress disorder, phobias, and selective mutism.

Why are anxiety disorders so prevalent?

There's no definitive answer, but I believe it's a combination of nature and nurture influences. Looking at environmental factors, our society has changed dramatically, becoming much faster paced and more complex. And family life is now more hectic and challenging than ever. As a key dynamic today, technology has had positive effects in reducing stress in some ways, but it has raised it in many other ways.

Our world is an increasingly anxious place. We have experienced 9/11, subsequent terrorist attacks, a financial crash, unthinkable school violence, devastating natural disasters, accelerated drug abuse, school bullying, more academically high-pressured kids, dramatic racial divides, and much more general tribulation. In short, familial, social, technological, economic, natural, and political forces have all stressed us out to the max—but these have also informed us about how to raise our kids and manage stress.

Certainly, we have advanced in diagnosing and treating anxiety, although most anxious kids receive no—or inadequate—treatment. Many families have been frustrated because various forms of therapy, however well meaning, and medication have not worked.

Family functioning is deeply affected when a child experiences anxiety. Parents are usually not prepared to help their anxious child, and dealing with an anxious child can be confusing. Parents may feel desperate as they search for effective guidance and support.

An Answer

The good news is that cognitive behavioral therapy (CBT) is an extremely useful approach for identifying and managing anxious thoughts and feelings. Through a family approach based on CBT (explored in depth in the book's first chapter), parents and their children can learn strategies together, creating teamwork and strengthening family bonds.

This book describes a proven approach—cognitive behavioral therapy— to help anxious kids while actively engaging parents in the process. Other books effectively address some important issues, but none presents a behaviorally grounded how-to strategy to confront these problems. Accordingly, with so many families crying out for help, I felt compelled to construct the CBT-based 7-Step TRAINOR Method as a simple and pragmatic way to find solutions.

This book puts the TRAINOR Method to work. It is written primarily for parents, to help them learn more about anxiety disorders and symptoms of child anxiety. It also gives a voice to these anxious children, who are often misunderstood. Families and mental health and related professionals all will find this approach beneficial.

The children and teenagers I have treated differ in many respects, but children with anxiety can all benefit from many common strategies and lessons learned from the step-by-step TRAINOR approach. These strategies are mapped out in the book through case studies based on my interactions with real patients and parents, though in some instances I provide a composite view of the sessions in an attempt to be more comprehensive and informative for readers. In most chapters I outline my meetings with parents and then with the kids; sometimes I see them separately and sometimes as a group, starting with a younger child's experience and continuing with an adolescent's case study. I describe the initial challenges, the strategy, and the results.

At the end of chapters 3–8 the reader will find the *DSM-5* criteria that are used in diagnosing a child with the anxiety disorder described in that chapter. The *Diagnostic and Statistical Manual of Mental Disorders* (DSM) is the standard catalog of mental disorders that mental health professionals in the United States refer to in making diagnoses; it includes a list of diagnostic criteria for every psychiatric disorder recognized by the U.S. healthcare system. (The *DSM-5,* which is the fifth edition of the manual, was published by the American Psychiatric Association in 2015.) Many anxious children do not meet the full criteria of a formal diagnosis but can benefit from the strategies outlined in this book. The *DSM* criteria are included for readers' information only. There is no expectation or even wish for parents to learn to diagnose or to practice diagnosing; diagnoses must be done by professional mental health providers who have expert training in diagnosis and treatment.

I focus on the most common anxiety problems and provide a fair amount of detail, since understanding the nuances is critical to success. I also provide information on additional resources, with the understanding that this therapy isn't a quick fix; although we expect positive results, the process of overcoming anxiety requires a commitment to work together as a team.

Those who share their experiences in this book represent the voices of my greatest teachers—the many children and parents I've worked with through the years. Each parent and child described in this book illuminates the experiences of wonderful children and loving families dealing with anxiety. The parents all have one thing in common: anxious children and a desire to help them.

I hope this book offers parents and professionals an understanding of anxiety in children and how to help anxious children overcome their problems.

....

Chapter 1

Fighting Anxiety

Applying CBT with a Step-by-Step Approach

As a therapist, I see many parents of anxious children who feel exhausted and isolated because their child seems happy in so many ways yet causes unbelievable chaos, confusion, and frustration at home—stressful reactions mostly hidden from the outside world. How can we best understand what it means when a child is anxious? Is there anything particular a parent can do when raising a child who has anxiety problems?

This chapter begins to explore these questions, providing an overview about anxiety and how children and parents can work together to treat it. I also discuss what to consider in using medication as part of the treatment. Finally, I address cognitive behavioral therapy (CBT) and introduce the 7-Step TRAINOR Method as a framework for successful outcomes. (The specifics of this step-by-step approach are illustrated in greater detail in chapter 2.)

I begin with a discussion of the biological bases of anxiety. Although understanding the scientific explanations of anxiety is not required in order to benefit from treatment, children and families are encouraged to be active partners on their therapy team, and healthcare providers should at least review this information with families.

Anxiety Overview and Biological Underpinnings

Anxiety is the most common psychiatric disorder among children and adolescents, with statistics suggesting epidemic levels: an estimated 12.3 percent of children have met the criteria for an anxiety disorder by the time they're in middle childhood, and up to 30 percent of all children and adolescents have been diagnosed with an anxiety disorder at some point.[1] Those numbers are astounding, considering that many anxious children may not meet the full criteria for a "disorder" but are still negatively affected by their irrational fears.

Anxiety doesn't go away with time; kids don't "outgrow" it. If anything, it tends to worsen over time. Anxiety can be normal at certain developmental stages, but when it persists, it can become problematic. Left untreated, it's likely to affect emotional, social, academic, and occupational functioning. Most people underestimate the impact of anxiety, not only in childhood but throughout life. Childhood anxiety has been shown to precede adult anxiety, alcohol and drug addiction, and poor physical health in young adulthood. For example, research shows that 35 to 45 percent of people struggling with alcohol and drug addictions also have an anxiety disorder. They may be "self-medicating" their anxiety with substance abuse.[2]

Anxiety is caused by biological vulnerabilities, chronic stress, traumatic life events, or some combination of these. And it runs in families. Anxious parents have a greater chance of having anxious children.[3] The nature versus nurture debate is ongoing, but the source of anxiety seems most often to be a combination of both. The cause of childhood anxiety is a complicated interplay of genetics, brain function, environmental stressors, and parenting styles.[4] The biological underpinnings of anxiety; the cognitive aspects, or the distorted thinking that comes with anxiety; and the dysfunctional reaction parents may have to their child's anxiety; all are important to understand.

Later in this chapter, I review the critical role that parents play in the development and treatment of anxiety as well as in its prevention. But overall, what is most important is that when parents learn how to raise a child who is anxious, they can make a huge difference in reducing the child's anxiety symptoms and in fostering healthy growth and development.[5]

Several parts of the brain constitute the "fear circuitry," which controls emotional regulation and the processing of fear. These include the amygdala, the ventromedial prefrontal cortex, and the anterior cingulate cortex, which I describe below. It's believed that anxious children may have structural as well as functional differences in these areas of the brain. Parents often feel their anxious child is simply "wired differently." Recent research on the anxious brain is proving parents to be right in some respects.[6]

The *amygdala* is almond shaped and located deep within the temporal lobe of the brain. The temporal lobe is involved in processing sensory input into meanings for the retention of visual memories, language comprehension, and emotion association. The amygdala is the part of the brain that controls the fear response. It processes and consolidates memories associated with emotional events. The amygdala imprints in the brain the reaction of synapses that elicit fear (synapses transmit and receive impulses from nerves). The amygdala can trigger release of stress hormones, which create the physical response of anxiety, including rapid heartbeat, sweating, stomach discomfort, shaking, and other panic symptoms. Increased activation in the amygdala along with possible structural differences have been identified in anxious children relative to children who don't suffer from anxiety.

When a child has an anxious reaction to an experience, the amygdala retains that memory of fear. This intense memory causes the child's extreme response to be maintained. Activation of the amygdala influences the strength of anxious, emotional memories and promotes fear conditioning.[7] This can explain what parents observe in their anxious child's automatic, intense, and irrational reaction when anxious. Parents will often say, "When she gets anxious, she can go from 0 to 100 in seconds." They are witnessing their child's automatic, poorly modulated fear response.

The *ventrolateral prefrontal cortex* modulates the activity of the amygdala and has also been shown to have increased activation in anxious children. This part of the brain attempts to provide emotional regulation and to process fear. It processes past emotional associations with events. When this function isn't working effectively, emotions may become confused, and the experience of fear can feel overwhelming. This explains why a child who becomes flooded with anxiety acts in a way that appears to her parents to be irrational and agitated.

The *anterior cingulate cortex* (ACC) processes cognitive and emotional information and the functional integration of both. It regulates blood pressure and heart rate and influences rational cognitive functions and modulation of emotional response to stimuli. MRIs (magnetic resonance images) have shown increased activation in this part of the brain too in anxious children.[8] When these three parts of the brain are not functioning well together, anxiety takes over. Parents often recognize their anxious child as having a "panic attack," with a rapid heartbeat and obvious physical symptoms of intense fear.

As we learn more about brain development, it appears that the brains of children with anxiety function differently from the brains of children without anxiety. Children with anxiety more easily become activated by fear, and their thinking quickly becomes irrational. They have trouble controlling their anxious feelings, and their bodies seem to experience stronger reactions to fear. This is all because of how their brains are "wired."[9]

It's important to consider this brain connection and remember that anxious children don't choose to be afraid; rather, they are likely experiencing intense anxiety because their brains are overactive in the areas that process fear. This brain processing likely has a genetic component, which is why some kids and parents are more anxious than others.

Overall, the brain is a powerful controlling organ that we know too little about, but we're learning more and more. We do know that, due to the brain's "wiring," anxious children have a distortion in their ability to perceive their surroundings and to process information. They tend to react to ambiguous stimuli as negative and interpret benign information as a threat. They see danger when there is no danger. They tend to be hypervigilant and automatically imagine that if something bad has even a remote chance of happening, it will happen. When anxious, their thinking becomes impulsive and distorted, causing them to feel fear when there is nothing to be afraid of. Their strong emotional reactions limit their ability to access and apply coping strategies.

When flooded with anxiety, anxious children feel the fear in their bodies because their overactive brains release stress hormones. This reaction is confusing for the children and causes more fear and distorted thinking, which in turn causes anxiety to spiral. This is also known as the "worry loop." It's real, and kids can get stuck in it, escalating their arousal and fear, quickly leading to a panic response, with rapid breathing, dizziness, stomach pain, nausea, shakiness, and often yelling and tears.

Different kids may respond differently when anxious. Some kids shut down and appear very frightened. They "implode" and may look frozen, with a "deer in the headlight" look. Other kids become emotionally dys-regulated when they're anxious, and they "explode." That's another way of saying they have angry tantrums. There's evidence that the neural mecha-nisms of emotional regulation are different in anxious kids. This can easily fool parents and others who expect a frightened child to be withdrawn and helpless looking, not kicking and screaming.

Understanding these tantrums as a child's version of a panic attack can change the response to them. Rather than responding with anger, it's more effective to try to help calm the child. When a child's brain is overactive in this manner, attempts to be rational or to discipline only escalate the anxiety.

Medication: When Is It Appropriate?

Medications are being prescribed for anxious children and adolescents now more than ever.[10] This is big business, with psychiatric medications bringing in billions of dollars for pharmaceutical companies. We are all influenced by this business, because pharmaceutical ads are everywhere. Unfortunately, too many kids are prescribed medication as a first line of treatment, without any therapy involved. In addition to the pharmaceutical companies, insurance companies also benefit from this practice because it's cheaper to medicate a child than it is to cover the cost of therapy. Parents are often reluctant to medicate their children, but when a medication is recommended by a professional, it can be hard to resist.

Research is incomplete on the long-term effect of these medications on children's developing minds and bodies. We do know, however, that children who take medications often experience side effects. And, perhaps most important, children treated with medication for anxiety may not be learning the strategies and skills that will help them manage their anxious feelings. The message is: a pill will take care of it.

Anxiety can be mild, moderate, or severe. In some cases of severe anxiety, medication can help a child function and access therapy. When a child is flooded with severe anxiety, learning and applying strategies can feel impossible. With medication, the anxiety can be reduced to facilitate learning.

So the caveat with medication is to proceed with caution and use medication as part of the treatment plan only when necessary and always in addition to therapy.

Cognitive Behavioral Therapy and the TRAINOR Method

Cognitive behavioral therapy (CBT) is an evidence-based treatment for child anxiety.[11] *Evidence based* means there's strong research proving its effectiveness in helping children significantly reduce their anxiety symptoms. In short, it's treatment that's been proved to work, even with very young children.[12] In addition, it has demonstrated long-term effectiveness, with the positive treatment effects maintained many years after the CBT treatment.[13] The cognitive part of the therapy involves changing the way a child thinks about irrational fears; the behavioral part engages the child in changing avoidant behavior.

The TRAINOR Method illustrated in this book applies CBT in a family-based approach that is individualized and engages both child and parents in the change process. Involving parents—not just through brief parent training, but through active engagement in working with their child—has been shown to be an effective treatment approach for anxious children. In addition to reducing children's anxiety, a CBT approach that involves parents improves family functioning.[14]

The TRAINOR Method simplifies and structures CBT in a manner that parents can use to help their anxious child. This therapy doesn't happen only in the therapist's office; it happens every day, with parents and teachers helping the anxious child apply and practice strategies and achieve goals to reduce anxiety. Applying CBT strategies has been shown to actually change the brain. We are learning more and more about brain *plasticity,* meaning the brain changes for the better with environmental influences such as CBT, and for the worse with exposure to trauma or chronic stress. Many clinical studies have shown that CBT changes the wiring of the brain. It changes dysfunctions in the nervous system. Through the technologies of positron emission tomography (PET) and functional magnetic resonance imaging (fMRI), by which we take pre- and post-CBT-treatment brain scans, dramatic brain changes have been proved to happen as a result of CBT. Feelings and behaviors involve specific brain circuits, and changes in thinking and behavior are associated with cerebral alterations.[15] This is exciting research that integrates neurobiology, psychopathology, neuropsychology, and psychotherapy.

Families are deeply affected by an anxious child and often seek treatment, desperate for guidance, because family functioning seems to have been turned upside down by the anxious child's symptoms. Working together, parents and children can learn strategies that increase understanding and promote change.

Parenting an Anxious Child: A Closer Look

Effective methods for parenting an anxious child may seem counterintuitive. The natural parenting response to a child who's exploding with anxiety is to want to take control and set limits. An anxious child is a child who needs to learn how to calm down and gain greater control of his thoughts and emotions. This is something the child has to learn through CBT, and parents can't do it for him. Reacting with anger only increases the child's arousal and explosive behavior. Attempting to talk to a child in this anxious state is also ineffective because the aroused brain interferes with the child's ability to be rational. When in fear mode, the anxious child's ability to solve problems and use coping strategies becomes impossible.

To avoid these explosive outbursts, parents often find themselves giving in or accommodating the anxiety. Parents "walk on eggshells," wanting to avoid major disruptions that can affect the whole family. This doesn't feel right for parents but often is necessary. When this happens, parents may feel angry and frustrated with their child and lose confidence in their ability to parent. In this situation, both parents and child are held hostage by anxiety.

When the child is imploding, rather than exploding, with anxiety, the child provokes a different response from parents. This child looks shut down, frozen, pale, and often sick. The instinctual response is to protect your child from pain. Yet this parenting style promotes avoidance behavior and accommodates the anxiety. Parental accommodation has been shown to cause more severe anxiety symptoms and longer term negative consequences for the child.[16]

When not confronted with anxiety-producing challenges, anxious children look very relaxed. This is what makes accommodation so tempting. For example, letting a scared child sleep with parents is disruptive but easier. The child goes to sleep peacefully, and everyone sleeps well. Not letting the child in the bed feels far more disruptive, with the child screaming in fear in the middle of the night, waking everyone up. Though everyone knows having a big kid in the parental bed isn't helpful in the long run because the child's fears aren't confronted, the drive to avoid the fear reactions and keep the peace so that everyone sleeps is very understandable. But again, the short-term gains usually lead to longer term, more severe problems with anxiety.[17]

Anxious parents are often described as overprotective in the literature, and this is interpreted as a causal factor in the development of a child's anxiety. An anxious parent, like an anxious child, has the tendency to see danger when there is none and to imagine all kinds of catastrophes happening. Helping an anxious child to change means that anxious parents have to change as well. Parents may be transmitting verbal and behavioral messages to their child that promote anxiety. This is the "nurture" aspect of the development of childhood anxiety. This parenting style, added to genetic tendencies passed down from parent to child, creates a combination that almost guarantees the development of severe childhood anxiety.[18]

Overprotective parenting and accommodating anxiety may not be a cause of anxiety so much as a reaction when parenting an anxious child. When how the child is wired is the primary cause of anxiety, accommodating feels like an automatic reaction. This is made most clear when parents of multiple children notice how differently they parent when challenged by their child who is anxious than they do when challenged by their child who is easygoing. Without an understanding of the biological underpinnings of anxiety, it's easy to blame parents. All children are not born equal when it comes to the genetic predisposition for anxiety. Terrific parents who are praised for their "calm child" are the same parents who can be harshly judged by others when their anxious child is acting out. Parents are often blamed, and feel blamed, when others witness their anxious child at her worst.

Fortunately, as noted before, CBT has been shown to be very effective in treating children with anxiety disorders. It focuses on changing the cognitive distortions of anxiety and the behavioral reactions children have to anxious feelings. Research consistently demonstrates that parents play critical roles in the development and transmission of anxiety in their children. Whether we lean toward nature or nurture, parents need to be very involved in treatment. They need to learn how to recognize when anxiety is playing a role in their child's thinking and behavior, and they need to learn to recognize their dysfunctional parental responses.

How Cognitive Behavioral Training and the TRAINOR Method Work

The TRAINOR Method helps parents feel more comfortable changing their parenting approach to promote exposure, instead of protection and avoidance. Parents are very engaged in the TRAINOR Method because they are the most important change agents for their anxious child. Anxiety for children is a daily, minute-to-minute, hour-to-hour experience. Parents live with their children and are in the unique position to promote their child's work toward making cognitive and behavioral changes every day. Anxious children need to apply specific CBT strategies daily to make a difference. It's this practice that changes the brain. For an anxious child, talking or playing with a therapist once a week is well meaning but not enough.

Anxiety is brain and behavior driven, and to change a child's thinking and behavior demands a more intensive approach. For children, this means parents must be actively involved with an approach that is reinforced and involves accountability. The TRAINOR Method guides parents and children to work together in this process of learning how to manage anxiety.

Involving parents also educates them about anxiety and the most effective parenting approaches for their child. Parents of anxious children are desperate to learn strategies that work. Even the smartest, most relaxed parents, when confronted with a very anxious child, often feel totally incompetent. Everything they think should work often doesn't. These parents are eager to learn how to help their anxious child calm down.

As noted before, CBT works by changing the way a child thinks (the cognitive part) and by changing how a child behaves in response to anxious feelings (the behavioral part). The two parts go hand in hand. If children think they're in danger, the smart thing is to avoid it. If a car is coming, and a child is in the middle of the street, he better get out of the way. When there's an anxiety disorder, kids feel like they're in danger when they're not. They want to run and avoid these feelings. But pushing through the experience, absorbing the anxious feelings, and experiencing that nothing bad happens help challenge these anxious thoughts. And changing anxious thinking and behaviors will change the brain and reduce the anxiety.

Denial and avoidance, which I address further in the next chapter, are the major defenses against anxiety. Kids have to learn to stop avoiding and to take on challenges step by step, knowing that with experience and practice, the anxious feelings will go away and will be replaced with positive feelings of mastery. This is the behavioral part of the therapy, and in many ways, the behavioral part of CBT is the most important. If a child understands there's nothing to be afraid of but continues to avoid anyway, change won't happen. Changing behavior reinforces that there's nothing to fear.

It's like the kid who can swim, standing at the edge of the diving board, afraid to jump. Understanding there's nothing to be afraid of, and talking about it over and over again, is fine but not enough. Taking that jump into the water and coming up, experiencing pride in overcoming fear, is what makes the difference. That behavioral change also makes a difference in the child's brain. Experiences change the brain, far more than thinking or talking about change does. Doing it, experiencing the challenge to anxiety, is far more powerful than talking about it. The CBT-based TRAINOR Method is effective because of the concrete behavioral goals that are agreed on and practiced by the child, with the support of her parents.

The anxious child has to do the work to get better, and parents have to learn how to set behavioral goals for their anxious children that are challenging but not overwhelming. Again, parents have to learn not to accommodate anxiety, even though accommodating feels like the best and sometimes only course of action. A child who never challenges her anxious feelings will continue to be afraid, and that fear will increase. As parents of anxious children, the message can't be "If it makes you uncomfortable, you don't have to do it." With the TRAINOR Method, the message is "If it makes you uncomfortable, we will break it down into steps, because there's nothing to be afraid of; you can do it, and it's very important that you do it."

The TRAINOR Method depends on parents acting as coaches with the "You can do it" attitude and the expectation that their child will push through the anxious feelings to function at a higher level.[19] Establishing cognitive and behavioral goals begins the change process. The TRAINOR Method stresses the importance of reasonable goals that are not forced on children but that both parents and child agree on. This promotes a collaborative approach to overcoming anxiety. Parents providing positive daily reinforcement strengthens the effectiveness of CBT treatment for the child.

To be sure, anxious children are scared children who feel a strong need to be in control, which makes them seem stubborn. Getting them to agree on goals that push them out of their comfort zone involves the use of incentives and rewards. They are being asked to do things that will initially make them feel anxious. This will feel uncomfortable. They are also being asked to gain self-control and not become so dysregulated. Learning how to calm down can be very hard work. Without incentives, this is a hard sell, and parents can't do this work for their child. Incentives motivate, and as the child begins to feel successful and less anxious, success builds on success, and the incentives often become less important for motivation.

The 7-Step TRAINOR Method recognizes that anxiety is not a child's problem alone; it affects the whole family. It's not a cookie cutter approach because every child and family is different, and anxiety comes in many forms and may be mild, moderate, or severe. Accordingly, this approach is individually tailored for each child and family. It engages parents in the treatment process with great respect for the role of parents in helping their child. Parents, as leaders of the family, become leaders in helping their anxious child become free of fear. This empowers parents to empower their children to live more full and productive lives, not burdened by the destructive, lifelong effects of untreated anxiety.

I invite you to learn more!

Chapter 2

Stepping Up to the Challenge

How the 7-Step TRAINOR Method Works

The 7-Step TRAINOR Method will guide you toward finding your way out of the grips of anxiety and regaining some peace of mind for your entire family.

TRAINOR is an acronym that aids you in remembering each of the seven steps:

Target
Rate
Agree
Identify
Note
Offer
Reinforce

In the first chapter, I provided general notes about cognitive behavioral therapy and how it is connected to the TRAINOR Method. In this chapter, I examine each of the seven steps and illustrate how they are applied to help anxious kids.

Denial

The TRAINOR Method starts by confronting the number-one defense against anxiety: denial. Both children and parents experience denial— an unconscious defense mechanism that often limits acknowledging the painful realities, thoughts, or feelings of dealing with anxiety or raising an anxious child. Parents adapt, or give in, to not rock the boat. As one parent described it: "We walk on eggshells, doing things—some that seem crazy—because we don't want to set her off. If we don't give in to her, she has a meltdown lasting an hour or more. We do these bizarre things—that we know other parents of kids her age don't do—to avoid a struggle."

You and your child will learn to work together to confront the denial. You will change how you think and respond to the anxiety invading your home.

This chapter details the seven steps of the TRAINOR Method to get you started.

TRAINOR Method Step 1: Target Anxious Thoughts and Behaviors

Target: To direct an action at something.

Begin by zooming in on your child's trouble areas, which will help you identify the stressors. Do this by noticing what precedes the reactive behaviors and considering two questions:

- What are the anxious thoughts?
- What are the anxious behaviors?

Moving from a place of denial to one of perspective, with the ability to back away and observe the problem, is a vital first step. This may not seem easy at first, and you may think, "But I am too frazzled at the moment to think about the anxious thoughts and behaviors." This is true: in the moment may not be the right time, but taking the time later to sort through the anxieties that create difficult behaviors will bring you one step closer to improvement. Until we face the fact that anxiety problems are not fixable by denial, wishful thinking, or hoping for different circumstances next time, the problems will likely persist.

The following is an example of how this worked for one family.

Ally and Steven came to talk about their 10-year-old daughter, Missy. Ally explained: "Missy is a great girl—loving, caring. She has lots of friends. We get compliments about her all the time. But she worries way too much about one thing: vomiting. The weird thing is she's probably thrown up twice in her life, yet this is her big fear. No matter what we tell her, it doesn't help."

Nobody enjoys the thought of vomiting, but for Missy, this fear immediately induced panic. Fear of vomiting is one of the most common phobias children and teens have. But Missy's fear of vomiting was so extreme, it literally made her sick, interfered with her life, and drove her family crazy.

Steven went on to explain how Missy expressed this fear. "She asks a zillion questions about getting sick," he said. "Every morning, it's 'Daddy, am I going to get sick at school today?' Every night, the same thing: 'Promise me I won't get sick.' If I don't promise her, she flips out. I feel like an idiot, but sometimes ten or fifteen times a day I find myself saying, 'You are not going to get sick; I promise you, you will not get sick.' It's senseless to us how worried she is about this."

Ally explained that instead of getting better, the problem was getting worse. "She goes to the nurse at school several times a day, worried about her stomach," Ally said. "If she eats a little too much at dinner and feels full, she panics. If she learns that anyone at school has been sick, she avoids them. The questions come all day long, at school and at home. She even has me come into the bathroom to check her bowel movements and make sure I don't see any signs of the stomach bug." Ally paused and looked away a second. "That's actually the first time I said this out loud," she continued. "I can't believe how ridiculous it sounds. She's 10 years old, and I check her poops; I think I may be losing it." Ally and Steven were finally facing the reality that these abnormal actions had become their "new normal." Anxiety had taken control not only of their daughter, but also of them.

In order to guide Missy, Ally and Steven first needed to consider their thoughts and behaviors in reaction to their daughter's behaviors. They had become sucked into this unsettling world ruled by anxiety. They hated it and found it frustrating. ("We argue about it; nothing we try works.") At times it made them feel angry. ("Stop with the questions. Go to bed. I've had enough!") They both experienced guilty feelings. ("She can't control herself, and she's so miserable over this. We should have more patience. We must be bad parents if we can't manage a 10-year-old.") They also felt terribly confused. ("We just don't know what to do anymore.")

We had to target their thoughts and behaviors—as well as Missy's—for change to occur. In fact, the whole family needed to learn how to help Missy manage her anxiety. Once they understood this, it would help them break through their denial and recognize the huge role they play in either helping her fight her anxiety or continuing to reinforce it.

Of course, Missy experienced denial, too. She believed strongly that her anxious thoughts were based on reality. She needed to challenge these thoughts, accept that she had to change, and most important, believe she was strong enough to control her worries about getting sick and vomiting, which induced panic.

What were Missy's anxious thoughts and behaviors? She avoided anything that might make her uncomfortable—a common reaction to anxious feelings. She sought reassurance from her parents for these anxious feelings every morning before school, every night before bed, and throughout the day at random times; at school, she frequently went to the nurse, and the nurse would call her parents. At first, her mother came to take her home, thinking she was sick. Soon, it became clear that her worries *made* her sick. Missy felt so anxious that she caused her stomach to hurt, which made her more worried about vomiting. Her mother stopped taking her home, but the nurse kept calling her to try to calm Missy down over the phone. Sometimes Missy felt okay after speaking to her mom, and she returned to class; other times, after talking to her mother, she cried more. The nurse would take her temperature, let her lie down, and eventually Missy would return to class. She would usually be back soon, however, and it would start all over again. She became a "frequent flier" to the nurse.

The more Missy asked about vomiting, the more she was stuck on it. She felt she needed reassurance to feel better, and this reassurance held a special power. Thoughts like these kept her reliant on frequent reassurance from others: "If Daddy doesn't promise, then I'll get sick." "I have to go to the nurse or I might vomit."

Another anxious behavior was worrying about food. She restricted her eating, afraid some foods would make her sick. And she stopped having breakfast. She said her stomach hurt every morning, and because she felt so scared she would vomit, she couldn't eat. Another behavior, which everyone dismissed as no big deal, was keeping a bucket next to her bed "just in case." If she needed to vomit in the night, she felt prepared. When I mentioned that this was not normal, her parents looked puzzled. They were so used to it that they never questioned it. It was a potent example of the family's denial.

Avoidance

The second major defense against recognizing and beginning to treat anxiety is avoidance. The parents' avoidance behaviors included all the abnormal things they did for her. They would do anything to avoid her meltdowns and to keep the peace—from checking her poops, to saying things over and over again "just the right way," to even being afraid to discipline her at all, for fear of setting her off. They hoped all this would just pass, even though it was getting worse. They found themselves focusing on how happy she could seem, laughing with her friends, playing soccer, and fooling around with her sister. She was even acting in a play. How could there be something wrong with her? They tried not to talk about it, except when the issues flared. Missy's worries about vomiting caused them to say, "We need help," but they continued to avoid doing anything about it, until they came for treatment.

Missy had many avoidance behaviors of her own. She stayed far away from anyone she thought might have been sick and even someone whose brother or sister was sick. She avoided hearing the word "vomit," freaking out and holding her hands over her ears if someone said the word. She also washed her hands too much to avoid getting germs on her hands. Missy's long list of avoidances included avoiding breakfast, spicy foods, and feeling full after eating—because then she would worry more.

Missy and her parents discussed openly her worries and her behaviors in reaction to her worries. They also described all the behaviors they were doing to reassure Missy when she was worried. It became clear how much Missy's anxiety was not only controlling her, but also controlling her parents. This is initially difficult to talk about, and reminding them that many, many families experience anxiety helped them feel less ashamed. After facing their denial and avoidance defenses, and analyzing the anxious thoughts and behaviors, Missy and her family were ready for Step 2.

TRAINOR Method Step 2: Rate the Anxious Behavior

Rate: Measure the value of something.

How do you begin to change all this? Where do you start? Once you have targeted the behaviors, it is important to have a rating system to chart progress.

One method for change that doesn't work is threats and punishments, as Ally, Missy's mom, experienced. "We tried getting her to stop all her talk and worries about sickness. We even threatened to punish her if she didn't stop," Ally began. "She just looked at us and started crying. She can't stop focusing on her fear of throwing up. We have no idea how to help her stop."

So together, we made a list of her anxious behaviors, and Missy then rated them, based on level of difficulty. She guided us to know where to start. She rated how hard it would be, on a scale of 0 (meaning it is easy) and 10 (meaning it is impossible), to

- Not ask Mom about getting sick 9
- Not ask Dad about getting sick 6
- Not ask Mom to check my poops 3
- Not sleep with a bucket 7
- Not avoid kids who have been sick 4
- Go on play dates 6
- Say the word vomit without holding my hands on my ears 5
- Watch a show where somebody vomits 7
- Let myself eat enough to feel full 6
- Go on sleepovers 9
- Not go to the nurse 9

Missy was clear about her hierarchy of difficulty. As her parents listened to her make and rate her list, they learned a lot and looked surprised by some of her responses. For instance, they had no idea the school nurse was so important to her. They had noticed Missy refusing play dates and sleepovers, but they'd had no idea it all came back to her fear of vomiting. Feeling afraid she would get sick at a friend's house, she stayed home. Ally was glad to learn that not asking her to check her poops was pretty easy for Missy, because her mother felt so ridiculous doing it. We all gained a good sense of the hardest and the easiest things for Missy and developed a much better understanding of her anxiety.

As you can see, the process of rating helps the child and parents understand the level of anxiety around particular anxious behaviors; it is a key tool for getting started. To think about goals for Missy to work on, we needed to understand which things were easier for her to work on and which were, at that time, too difficult.

TRAINOR Method Step 3: Agree on Challenges to Work On

Agree: Have the same opinion about something; concur.

Anxious children often do not want to work on changing the anxious behaviors they have rated: it feels too difficult. Easing them into it with gentle empowerment and excitement makes it easy.

In Missy's case, she felt afraid. She looked around her, anticipating that all the grownups in the room, including this *doctor*, would now force her to do things she felt way too scared to do. Like a kid at the edge of the diving board for the first time, scared to jump, she did not want to be pushed.

I started by saying, "We'll fight this step by step. You'll be the leader of the fight, and we're all part of your team."

Missy broke into a smile, looked at her parents, and felt a bit of power. She had never been the leader before with her parents. Then I mentioned that she would earn prizes doing this hard work, and her smile grew. She started to get excited, imagining what those prizes could be.

We looked at her working list together. The easiest thing was not asking Mom to check her poops. She had been asking her mom to do this at least four or five times a week. Every day she did not ask, she earned 1 point, and when she went seven days in a row without asking anyone to check her poops, she earned a bonus 5 points.

Not avoiding someone who had been sick was also not too difficult. Talking to a child who was back at school after being sick, or even touching them or their things, gained her another 5 points.

Not going to the nurse was a big one, rated very high. Her parents felt urgency about this one, because Missy missed a lot of class time. We usually start with the lower numbers and work our way up gradually to the harder things, but Missy's mom took a chance and asked if she was ready to work on staying in class and not going to the nurse. The mood in the room changed immediately. Missy hesitated. Tears welled up in her eyes. She looked at her parents with a mixture of fear and anger. A meltdown fast approached. The thought that we would say she could never go to the nurse overwhelmed her. She needed to know we would not force her to do something she was not ready to do. She felt she needed those visits to the nurse.

The more you push an anxious child too far, the more they push back with great force. Remember the kid at the edge of the diving board? Try to push him, and he will push back, turn around, and walk off the board angry, without jumping. Too many parents of anxious children know this battle too well, a battle you will never win.

I quickly chimed in and told Missy we would not take away her visits to the nurse. She was the leader of this team; we were there to help and support her. I also reminded her that the harder the work, the bigger the prize. She calmed down a bit. Prizes can be a great mood shifter. We discussed how often she went to the nurse. She told us she went at least once a day, sometimes four or five times a day. Her parents looked surprised and concerned. No wonder her grades had slipped so quickly. Not going to the nurse at all, at this point, would be too hard. By establishing this baseline, however, we figured out how to choose a challenging goal that would not overwhelm her. We broke it down: 10 points for not going to the nurse at all in a day, 5 points for going once, 2 points for going twice, and 0 points for going three or four times. Missy agreed. We couldn't set the goals too high, or she would fail; too low, and she would earn points without challenging her anxiety—making no progress.

We reviewed our plan all together so it was clear. She would work on not asking for her poops to be checked, cutting back on her visits to the nurse, and not avoiding anyone who had been sick. I asked her if she also wanted to work on anything else. Her look of fright said it all. We all agreed that this was enough to start. Working intensely on a few goals is better than trying to work on too many at once. If a child is overwhelmed by the goals in the beginning, effort is diminished. The child feels defeated before the work has even started.

TRAINOR Method Step 4: Identify and Teach Strategies to Practice

Identify: Establish or indicate who or what.

Now Missy and her parents knew what she would work on, but that was not enough. They needed to know how to do this—easier said than done. I explained to Missy that lots of kids get worries and have to learn to fight them and get rid of them. I explained to her that there are two kinds of worries: real worries and silly worries. Real worries are like when she is in the middle of a street and a car is coming. That is a real worry. She needs to get out of the street. If she has trouble at school and can't get help, that is a real worry. She needs to talk to someone and ask for help. These are problems that can be solved.

Silly worries are worries that lots of kids get when there is no danger. Some kids worry about aliens or monsters. Her silly worry is about throwing up. She is not silly; her worries are silly. She needed to reframe them by changing the way she thought about her worries.

Missy needed to remember that her worry about vomiting was a "silly worry." When she started thinking about it, she needed to refocus her attention on something else—to let it go and not be stuck on it. I suggested that her thoughts not be, "Don't think those scary thoughts about vomiting." Instead, I suggested she think, "Those thoughts are silly, not important. I want to think about other things." She began learning how to "talk back" to the anxiety.

We made a list of what she could focus on when she started to get the silly worries—how she could "change the channel in her head" off the worry channel. When home, she could listen to music, and she loved singing. She could make her own special calm-down playlist of songs and sing along. It's difficult to be worried and singing at the same time. We made a list of all the relaxing activities she could choose from when she began worrying about vomiting. She loved to read, draw, make up stories, ride her bike, and make special snacks. When she started to get the silly worry about vomiting and used this list to change her channel, she earned another 5 points.

What about at school? Missy needed to remember the vomiting worry as a silly worry and focus on what was going on around her: listening to the teacher, participating in class, talking to her friends at lunch, or keeping her attention on what is important at school, not on the silly worries.

We discussed how everybody's behavior would change to fight the anxiety and not be ruled by it. For Missy to get better, she had to first feel uncomfortable and experience a manageable level of distress. Her parents had to learn to do things that are counterintuitive for parents. As parents, from the time our newborn is placed in our arms, we have an instinct to protect and shelter our child from pain. Parenting anxious children demands the opposite response: we must support our children to push through their discomfort to get to the other side. We help our children learn to push themselves, even when it feels difficult, knowing that those anxious feelings will go away.

Protecting and sheltering your anxious child fuels the anxiety and makes it worse. An anxious child who is too comfortable is limited by the anxiety—her world will become smaller and smaller over time.

We discussed how Mom and Dad could help. They could remind Missy that she could meet her goals, praise her for her accomplishments in fighting the silly worries, and, of course, provide the rewards.

Not talking to her about the worries is important. We agreed, specifically, not to talk about her poops. If Missy forgot and asked, her mother could say "silly worry" as her reminder. If Missy felt worried, she could pick from her list of options to "change the channel" in her head. Her mother would avoid the repetitive conversation about how her poops are fine, that she is not going to vomit, and so on. Talking about her worries with Missy would only model that they were something she needed to talk about, something important. This would give Missy's worries too much attention and bring Missy and her parents back into the worry loop of "But Mom, what if . . . I need you to . . . It could be true . . . How do you know?" Such conversation rapidly escalates until Mom is once again staring down into a toilet bowl looking at perfectly normal poops, assuring her child she is not sick. Anxiety wins again, and everyone feels defeated. Instead, Missy and her parents had to learn, "No talking about it—silly worry—move on." Every time Missy did this, she would earn more points. Missy and her parents agreed to this plan and felt optimistic that they could now work together to help her manage her anxiety.

In addition, exposing herself to her fear is also very important to desensitize her to her fear of vomiting, which for Missy will include saying "vomit" and "throw up" and watching videos of people vomiting and rating her anxiety level until it goes down to zero. This graduated exposure would significantly help reduce her anxious response to vomiting.

TRAINOR Method Step 5: Note and Chart Progress Made

Note: To notice or pay particular attention to.

Once the wheels are set in motion, the next step is to note the desired actions and create a chart as a means of tracking results toward goals.

Missy and her parents made a chart that included what Missy was working on. She made her chart with her parents and decorated it. This was her chart, made in a way that she and her family deemed easiest to use. Some families use paper or poster board; others prefer the computer, an iPad, or a calendar. Whatever is clear, visual, simple, and easy for the family to use works best. Missy's chart, which they hung in the kitchen on the refrigerator, looked like this:

Missy Silly Worry Chart

- ❑ No checking P [code for poops in case non–family members might see the chart]
- ❑ Nurse: No? Yes? How many times?
- ❑ Not avoiding kids who have been sick
- ❑ Changing the channel in my head by picking from my activity list

Next we created another chart using a calendar format, because Missy needed to work on reducing her anxiety every day. Missy found a calendar on the computer and copied her list of worries onto every day on the calendar. Then she printed the calendar out. Every day that she did something from her list, she checked it off. Under the check, she gave it a number, 0 to 10, to show how hard it was. The more she practiced, the lower the numbers went, measuring how her anxiety decreased. Next, she recorded how many points she had earned for that worry on that day.

She and her parents chose a time each day to go over her points earned and add them all up. This kept the process positive and reminded her to keep working at her goals and not slip back. The first two weeks of Missy's calendar looked like the illustration on pages 28 and 29.

This wasn't always easy, of course. Some days the process went smoothly; some days Missy needed a boost, which was usually as simple as reviewing her rewards. And on days when her parents were busy with work issues or just typical active family life, they needed to force themselves to make time to sit with Missy and review the day. Their motivation? The baby steps of progress they were beginning to observe. Missy's motivation? The points and the powerful feelings of accomplishment. She was very proud of herself.

TRAINOR Method Step 6: Offer Incentives to Motivate

Offer: To present for acceptance or rejection.

As families proceed with the steps, the reward system needs to be carried out, to be sure the message is clear that prizes will come. Of course, for the parents, the reward is the child's changing behaviors, but the behavior changes may fall apart without carrying out the actual offers made when setting up the chart.

What do all these points mean for a child or adolescent? What can they cash them in for?

The younger the child, the quicker they need the rewards. Most children need a reward within a week of working hard. Some kids are motivated to work for something large. If the reward is too far in the future, it becomes abstract and not motivating; however, they can "bank" their points for something large and, in the meantime, receive smaller things along the way.

Missy and her parents agreed on prizes, which do not have to be purchased items but can also be activities or privileges; this can help alleviate concerns about spending money on rewards. The prizes can even replace treats that in the past did not have to be earned. Now, when Missy wanted a treat, instead of just getting it, she earned it through this hard work.

Missy's Silly Worry Calendar

How hard? Rate each worry on a scale of 0 to 10, with 10 the hardest.

How many points?

Not checking P: Every day without asking = 1 point; 7 days in a row without asking = bonus 5 points.

Talking to a child who was back at school after being sick, or even touching them or their things = 5 points.

Not going to the nurse at all in a day = 10 points; going once = 5 points; going twice = 2 points; going three or four times = 0 points.

Changing the channel in her head by picking from list = 5 points.

Missy's total points for this month: ___

Sunday	Monday	Tuesday	Wednesday	Thursday	Friday	Saturday
1	**2**	**3**	**4**	**5**	**6**	**7**
☐ Not checking P How hard? ___ How many points? ___	☐ Not checking P How hard? ___ How many points? ___	☐ Not checking P How hard? ___ How many points? ___	☐ Not checking P How hard? ___ How many points? ___	☐ Not checking P How hard? ___ How many points? ___	☐ Not checking P How hard? ___ How many points? ___	☐ Not checking P How hard? ___ How many points? ___
☐ Not avoiding kids who have been sick How hard? ___ How many points? ___	☐ Nurse: No? Yes? How many times? ___ How hard? ___ How many points? ___	☐ Nurse: No? Yes? How many times? ___ How hard? ___ How many points? ___	☐ Nurse: No? Yes? How many times? ___ How hard? ___ How many points? ___	☐ Nurse: No? Yes? How many times? ___ How hard? ___ How many points? ___	☐ Nurse: No? Yes? How many times? ___ How hard? ___ How many points? ___	☐ Not avoiding kids who have been sick How hard? ___ How many points? ___
☐ Changing the channel in my head by picking from my activity list How hard? ___ How many points? ___	☐ Not avoiding kids who have been sick How hard? ___ How many points? ___	☐ Not avoiding kids who have been sick How hard? ___ How many points? ___	☐ Not avoiding kids who have been sick How hard? ___ How many points? ___	☐ Not avoiding kids who have been sick How hard? ___ How many points? ___	☐ Not avoiding kids who have been sick How hard? ___ How many points? ___	☐ Changing the channel in my head by picking from my activity list How hard? ___ How many points? ___
Today's total points: ___	☐ Changing the channel in my head by picking from my activity list How hard? ___ How many points? ___	☐ Changing the channel in my head by picking from my activity list How hard? ___ How many points? ___	☐ Changing the channel in my head by picking from my activity list How hard? ___ How many points? ___	☐ Changing the channel in my head by picking from my activity list How hard? ___ How many points? ___	☐ Changing the channel in my head by picking from my activity list How hard? ___ How many points? ___	Today's total points: ___
	Today's total points: ___	Today's total points: ___	Today's total points: ___	Today's total points: ___	Today's total points: ___	

8	9	10	11	12	13	14
☐ Not checking P How hard? — How many points? —	☐ Not checking P How hard? — How many points? —	☐ Not checking P How hard? — How many points? —	☐ Not checking P How hard? — How many points? —	☐ Not checking P How hard? — How many points? —	☐ Not checking P How hard? — How many points? —	☐ Not checking P How hard? — How many points? —
	☐ Nurse: No? Yes? How many times? How hard? — How many points? —	☐ Nurse: No? Yes? How many times? How hard? — How many points? —	☐ Nurse: No? Yes? How many times? How hard? — How many points? —	☐ Nurse: No? Yes? How many times? How hard? — How many points? —	☐ Nurse: No? Yes? How many times? How hard? — How many points? —	
☐ Not avoiding kids who have been sick How hard? — How many points? —	☐ Not avoiding kids who have been sick How hard? — How many points? —	☐ Not avoiding kids who have been sick How hard? — How many points? —	☐ Not avoiding kids who have been sick How hard? — How many points? —	☐ Not avoiding kids who have been sick How hard? — How many points? —	☐ Not avoiding kids who have been sick How hard? — How many points? —	☐ Not avoiding kids who have been sick How hard? — How many points? —
☐ Changing the channel in my head by picking from my activity list How hard? — How many points? —	☐ Changing the channel in my head by picking from my activity list How hard? — How many points? —	☐ Changing the channel in my head by picking from my activity list How hard? — How many points? —	☐ Changing the channel in my head by picking from my activity list How hard? — How many points? —	☐ Changing the channel in my head by picking from my activity list How hard? — How many points? —	☐ Changing the channel in my head by picking from my activity list How hard? — How many points? —	☐ Changing the channel in my head by picking from my activity list How hard? — How many points? —
Today's total points: —	Today's total points: —	Today's total points: —	Today's total points: —	Today's total points: —	Today's total points: —	Today's total points: —

Note: The TRAINOR method works best when the child can see the difficulty level going down and the points going up.

Missy decided she would like to earn

- a special doll
- a sleepover with two friends
- being able to choose what the family would eat for dinner (within reason)
- having breakfast on the weekend alone with Dad
- an iTunes gift card
- an ice cream sundae

She and her parents agreed on how many points she needed for each prize. Missy's doll was worth 250 points, but every 20 points she earned got her a smaller prize. Missy was excited, and the process of working hard doing so many things that initially felt uncomfortable was actually manageable. She could do it!

TRAINOR Method Step 7:
Reinforce Progress and Increase Challenges

Reinforce: to strengthen by additional assistance, material, or support.

After a couple of weeks, Missy's calendar was all filled in. She'd earned prizes, and she felt excited to show me how many points she'd earned. We looked at her accomplishments. Not having Mom check poops was now easy, rated a 0, down from an initial rating of 3. Zero meant we could cross it off the list—she did it!

In the beginning, not going to the nurse was difficult, but after a while, she'd earned more days of maximum points for not going to the nurse at all. She rated that behavior a 2, down from an initial rating of 7; it was still a bit hard, but so much better.

Not avoiding kids who have been sick was another 0, down from a 4—she crossed that off the list. Missy was making great progress. What to work on next? We needed to increase her challenges.

She agreed to work on not asking Dad about getting sick. If she slipped and asked, she agreed Dad could say "silly worry" to remind her to let it go and move on. When it felt difficult, she would pick from her calm-down list. Every day that she did not ask Dad about getting sick, she would earn 5 points; every day that she asked but could stop and move on, she earned 3 points. And if she really needed him to give her reassurance because she felt so worried, he would, but she then would receive no points. She agreed.

Saying the word "vomit" without covering her ears still challenged her. She hated that word. Every day that she worked on saying the word "vomit" over and over, she earned 2 points. The more she did it, however, the quicker she would improve; exposure works so well with scenarios like this.

We agreed that Missy would keep working on not going to the nurse, but now she would earn her points by not going at all for five days in a row. She agreed to that challenge. She also agreed to go on play dates with her friends, a step in the direction of being able to do sleepovers again, since social isolation is often a symptom of anxiety and an important area to work on.

Missy now had a new chart, new work to be done fighting the anxiety, and more points and prizes to be earned.

Missy's parents came to meet with me privately a few times during these weeks to talk about their changing role and behaviors. They wanted to understand more about anxiety and how to help Missy. They also talked to me about her sister, who had some anxiety problems as well. When there are siblings involved, I often recommend that the siblings get a chart so that they can be working on things too. Since anxiety tends to run in families, often more than one child in a family has anxiety. If the other siblings are not anxious, there is always something they can work on, from making their bed to doing their homework without a fuss. This reinforces the message that every kid has something to work on and normalizes this process. It also discourages jealousy from the other siblings over getting prizes. As Missy's parents have demonstrated, the TRAINOR Method's seven steps provide a process for parents to leap out of their out-of-control zones and into a new and guided means of helping their child and themselves. It helped them move from feeling powerless and controlled by their child's anxiety to feeling united as a family empowering her to exercise control.

Next Steps

Missy continues to work hard and is now doing sleepovers with friends. She has an overnight school trip she wants to go on, however, and it's making her feel scared. We are discussing strategies, and this is giving her the confidence she needs to meet this goal and go with her friends. Her parents are also learning how to help her sister, Grace, with her anxiety, which is very different. Grace is relaxed in many ways but worries way too much about schoolwork. We are all working together to help both children feel free of anxiety.

Chapter 3

Daytime, Bedtime, Worry, Worry

Generalized Anxiety Disorder

All kids worry, but some kids worry to the extreme. Kids with generalized anxiety disorder (GAD) have worries that are more pervasive and persistent than others. They often think in terms of "What if . . . ?" They are highly sensitive to thinking that if something bad happens to someone, anywhere in the world, it could easily happen to them, or to their family. The natural response, to reassure them, leads to more anxiety and more "What if . . . ?"

Children with GAD have trouble keeping things in perspective. Parents intuitively know that these kids can't handle watching the news and often try to protect them from hearing anything "bad." They know it will start them worrying, which can be distressing and hard to stop. Once children with GAD get stuck on a worry, they may have trouble sleeping, and their fears can become so intense that they have crying meltdowns and are difficult to soothe. They get caught up in a "worry loop" of repeating the same "what ifs," and it can be hard to get out of this cycle.

Kids with GAD usually want to know exactly what to expect in their day-to-day life. When things become unpredictable, they seem unable to cope. Flexibility, change, and failure create extreme discomfort for them. As a result, getting them to engage in new activities can be difficult, and getting them to stick it out and not quit can seem impossible. Uncertainty can be hard for them to tolerate, and learning new things involves risk and possible failure.

These feelings can feel too overwhelming for kids with GAD to bear. They are often driven by perfectionism, and when engaged in learning, they quickly become self-critical. As we know, learning involves the opposite of perfectionism. We have to work and struggle, and we often make mistakes as we learn. When faced with challenges, kids with GAD become filled with anxious thoughts, including, "I'm not as good as everyone else. Kids will make fun of me, and I can't do it. This is too hard. I hate it. I don't want to do it." Kids never say, "I don't want to do it because it makes me feel too anxious." They say, "I don't like it. I hate doing that, and you can't make me do it." So parents are faced with a dilemma: they want their kids to participate in activities, but they don't want to force them to do things they don't like.

How can you force your child to do something he hates, especially considering that avoidance is the number-one defense against anxiety? Anxious children often avoid doing after-school activities or worse, refuse to go to school.

These kids may "hate" almost everything except staying home riveted to a screen. When that's the case, anxiety is making their choices for them. Screens and snacks become their companions and their preferred after-school activities. They are often most comfortable at home, eating the limited foods they like, and playing games or watching videos. Kids with GAD are often labeled "picky eaters," "homebodies," "gamers," "shy," or "just not into sports."

Kids with GAD often worry excessively about school performance. Their parents say they don't pressure them about grades, but the children seem to be internally driven to be perfect, which translates into getting perfect grades. This can cause them to spend way too much time on homework. They may make a simple homework assignment into a much bigger deal. When homework has to be perfect, it can take twice as long as it should. Anxiety about homework often leads to meltdowns. Some kids worry too much about tests, so the night before a test can be tense. Even when they are great students, anxious kids worry about failing. All this is usually happening in the evening, when everyone is tired—a recipe for an ugly scene. The more kids get anxious, the less they can focus on their work. Parents often dread homework time because of the stress it causes.

Kids with GAD may also have physical symptoms, most frequently headaches and stomachaches. Pediatric gastroenterologists are usually aware that a large proportion of their patients struggle more with anxiety than with any significant gastrointestinal problem. These physical symptoms often become the focus of parents' attention, with frequent visits to doctors and medical test after test coming back normal. Being physically sick also becomes a reason to avoid anxiety-producing activities.

Again, parents are in a dilemma: "How can I push her to go to school when she's sick?" Being sick may be a way for a child with GAD to defend against anxious feelings. And anxiety can actually make kids sick. The stomach and the brain are closely tied together. Kids may have stomach pain and may even vomit, but the worries are causing the pain, not an illness. Reducing the anxiety reduces the pain.

Kids may also have trouble sleeping, because at night, when all is quiet, there is more time to worry. Children with GAD need their sleep, exercise, and a healthy diet, or their symptoms can worsen. Knowing this can be frustrating for parents because getting kids with GAD to calm down and do the healthy things they need to do can be so difficult. Sleeping issues and eating problems often go hand and hand with anxiety.

Many of the above issues manifested themselves in the experiences described below.

Mike and Sarah's Story

Mike and Sarah came to me because they were very concerned about Lily, their 9-year-old daughter. Sarah spoke first. "Lily is a great little girl, but she worries all the time about everything. She's always been like this, but lately it's getting worse, and we don't know what to do to help her. I'm at my wits' end. She's a kid. She should be happy. She's a great student, but she worries every time there's a test. When she's studying the night before a test, she often ends up crying and screaming over the littlest thing. The strange thing is, she always gets fine grades. She also worries about her friends not liking her, but she has a good group of girls who always seem happy to play with her."

Sarah paused, then continued. "Her big worry, every night, is someone's going to come in our house and . . . I don't know what. Hurt her? Kidnap her? She doesn't say. She can't sleep in her bed. This has always been a problem with her, but now she's so old, and it's impossible to get her in her bed. Her room is at the top of the stairs, and she thinks this 'bad guy' will come into the house and get to her first. She seems terrified, so she sleeps with us every night. I know it sounds crazy, but within minutes, she goes right to sleep in our bed. We live in a safe neighborhood, have an alarm system, and our dog barks at everything. It doesn't matter to her. No matter how many times we tell her she's safe, she can't seem to get it through her head. It's always 'What if . . . ?' from her, no matter what we say. It can get ridiculous."

Sarah seemed exasperated. "Last night it was 'What if someone comes in, and the alarm doesn't work, and he gets the dog to be silent, and he's so quiet he doesn't wake you up, and he comes up the stairs and into my room?' It can go on and on. There's no getting through to her. Some nights she seems to almost have a panic attack if we try to make her stay in her bed, as if she's in total danger of being attacked."

Mike then jumped in. "She sleeps with you. I have to find a bed to sleep in; I usually end up in her bed or on the couch. It's ridiculous, but we all need our sleep." Sarah continued. "Another thing, I don't know if it's all related, but she has temper tantrums like a 2-year-old. She's almost 10—way too old for this behavior. She gets herself so worked up sometimes, she becomes hysterical, and there's no talking to her. We've tried punishing her, talking to her, ignoring her—nothing works. It's usually before we have to go somewhere, like her soccer games or practices, or in the morning before school. The littlest thing causes her to explode. This morning it was that she wanted to wear a short-sleeve shirt, and it's thirty degrees outside. That caused a screaming fit for almost a half hour. We barely made it to school on time.

"I can't tell you how disruptive this is for the whole family. Her little brother runs away scared when she gets like this. Then once she's out the door and goes to school or to her sports, wherever, she is this normal, happy girl for the most part. Change is hard for her to handle, and it's not summer anymore—she has to wear warm clothes."

Mike added, "She's always complaining of a stomachache and asking to go to the doctor. We have taken her to the doctor many times, and the pediatrician says there's nothing wrong with her. Lately she has been going to the school nurse and calling to get picked up. If we pick her up, as soon as she gets home, she's fine. Is she making this up, or is her anxiety really making her sick? This is so frustrating. We both work and can't keep missing work over this."

Sarah nodded, then said, "I know we're telling you all these bad things, but Lily is a terrific kid, kind, sensitive, and sweet. When you meet her, you'll see. She's adorable. No one would imagine this same girl acts so scared and out of control at home. I always get the best reports from teachers, coaches, and other parents. In fact, her teacher told me, at the last conference, she wishes all the kids were like her. I bit my tongue, but I felt like saying, come and live with us for twenty-four hours and you might change your mind!"

"I must admit, I lose my patience with her," said Mike. "Nothing I do seems to work. If I try to joke about it, she gets mad. If I try to talk seriously with her about how crazy these fears are, she starts screaming at me that I don't understand. If there's something to worry about, she will find it. Lily has had a very stable home. No big changes in her life."

Then Mike added an interesting wrinkle to the discussion: "She reminds me of my mother. When I was a kid learning to swim, my mom talked endlessly about drowning and how I needed to learn to swim, not because it was fun, but so I wouldn't drown. I would go to the playground, and she would imagine me falling off the jungle gym and cracking my skull open."

He then looked at his wife and said, "Honestly, you know, that's the way Mom is, and sometimes Lily seems like mini-Mom. Seeing this anxiety in Lily drives me crazy. I love my mother, but she's a stress machine. Lily is not my mother, I know. I just don't want her growing up to be anxious like my mom. What can we do to help her? What did we do wrong? We have a younger son, and he's just the opposite. Nothing bothers him. Why can't she be more like him? What really upset both of us was the other night, after I tried and failed once again to get her to sleep in her own bed, she had a meltdown, crying and screaming, and at one point, she said she wished she was dead. To hear my little girl say such a thing really tore me apart. We know we need help with this."

Clearly, it sounded like Mike's mother had anxiety issues, and I explained to Mike and Sarah that anxiety is often genetic. I then asked them more about family history. Sarah laughed and said, "Aha! She gets this from your side."

Mike laughed too. "Yes, it's my fault . . . but let's talk about your family. Your father, for starters!"

Sarah laughed again. "Yes, he's right. My father was always a worrier and very overprotective of me and my sisters. We needed to sneak around to go out with our friends, knowing he would want us to stay home. We were all so glad to go to college and get freedom. My mother was great, but my aunt had a lot of problems. I remember she would just stay in her house and not go out. I could never understand it. She even had groceries delivered, and she never came to family functions. I think I met her once when she was sick and my mom brought some soup to her. My mom would say, 'She's just a homebody,' whatever that meant. Could that have been anxiety?"

She then smiled at Mike and said, "Okay, maybe it's not all your fault."

Mike said, "I guess the poor kid has no chance with our genes. She gets it from both sides, and we just need to know how to help her. I love my mother, but I don't want Lily growing up with my mother's anxiety. There has to be a way we can prevent that and help her."

I reassured them that there was a way. We needed to hear from Lily.

Lily's Story

Lily did seem like the sweet, engaging child her parents described, but she was obviously conflicted, and she echoed many of her parents' comments while meeting with me.

"I worry about lots of things. I can't help it. My biggest worries are at night. I'm so scared someone could come into the house and into my room. I can't sleep in my room; I keep hearing noises and think someone's coming. I can't stand it. I need to run into Mom and Dad's bed. Then I feel safe and can sleep. I know other kids my age sleep alone, and I don't want anyone to know I sleep with my parents. At night, when it's dark out, I can't even go upstairs when everyone else is downstairs. I get so scared. I feel like someone could be hiding up there. I hate when it's dark."

She shuddered a bit, then continued. "I have other worries too. I worry about school all the time. Tests are the worst. I hate tests. I worry that I could fail or forget everything, and it makes me so scared. My teacher is nice, but what if she gets mad at me? And my friends—sometimes I think they don't like me. Sometimes I think I have no friends, and I get so upset. I know I have friends, but what if they are mad at me? My mom wants me to have a birthday party, and I want to, but I'm scared no one will come, or if they come, they won't have fun. What if no one comes to my party? I told her I don't want a party."

Lily caught her breath. "Then there's sports. My mom and dad want me to play, and I like soccer and basketball, but I worry. What if I mess up and everyone sees it? Maybe they won't want me on the team anymore. Before the games and the practices, I get so upset sometimes, my stomach starts to hurt, and I just wish I could stay home. I don't know why, but before I leave the house, everything just makes me crazy, and I start screaming and crying. I just get so upset and angry. I want to stay home. My parents get so mad at me when I'm like this. I know it's bad, but I can't help it. I don't know why it happens. Once I get to soccer and start playing, it's fun, and I feel so happy. One of my coaches even said I was a great soccer player."

Lily began feeling more comfortable as she continued: "My parents tell me to never watch the news. It scares me to hear about bad things. I can't stop thinking these bad things could happen to me. When it gets cloudy out, I start to worry about things like hurricanes and tornadoes, and sometimes, I just don't want to go outside. If there are big clouds, I get too scared. I have a lot of things that make me worry.

"I know sometimes I get really angry and upset, especially at night or before tests. I always feel so sorry after. My mom understands, I think, but my dad, he can be mean. Mom always lets me in their bed and doesn't get so mad, but Dad can get angry. He says 'Lily, you have to go in your room. Don't be silly. You can do it.' When I get upset, he tells me to stop crying. I wish I could! It's not that easy. I don't want to be like this. He doesn't understand. I'm really scared. Why am I like this? Nobody understands that I can't change this; it's just the way I am. My parents brought me to another doctor, and she was nice, and we played games. They stopped taking me because they said nothing was getting better. I can't change this, and I want everyone to leave me alone. I don't want anything to change. There's not such a big problem."

It appeared that Lily wanted help but was convinced she couldn't change. This was a girl who hated failure and had no confidence she could get help. We were now ready to start working together and giving her more confidence in her ability to gain self-control and learn how to manage her worries.

Step 1: Target Anxious Thoughts and Behaviors

Not surprisingly, when Lily and her parents came together for the next session, she made it clear that she wanted no part of continued therapy. When she came into my office, she made no eye contact, sat really close to her mother, and whispered to her, "When can we go home?" She then took one of the pillows on my couch and put her head behind it. She was showing me how mad and oppositional she could be. Her father just looked down at the floor, and her mother's face started getting red. It was like both parents were saying, "Here we go again. What are we supposed to do?"

Her mother then said, "It was a huge battle to get her here." Then she turned to Lily and said in a stern voice, "Lily, don't be rude."

With that, Lily started crying. We were off to a horrible start.

Lily was like many kids with anxiety who are high functioning and, as a result, hate feeling so helpless and out of control. Lily wanted to be the girl teachers love and friends invite to parties, the girl who is a great athlete. She didn't want to be the weird girl who needed to see a therapist. She felt ashamed and hopeless about this part of herself, her anxious self. She was angry about having these problems, and her anger was directed at her parents and anyone who wanted to help her with her anxiety. Instead, she needed to learn to get angry at her worries so that she could work to be free of them. She needed help to integrate her strengths and her struggles. She needed to learn that one doesn't negate the other, and we all have both. After all, Lily was smart, athletic, popular, and, at times, struggling with painful anxiety. She needed to know that lots of great kids have these same worries and that she would learn how to free herself from them.

To normalize her experience, we talked about how many kids struggle with worries. I let her know that I see other kids from her school. She looked surprised. She had thought she was the only kid in the world, never mind in her school, who had worries.

She perked up. "Who else in my school comes here?"

I explained that I couldn't tell her because it's private. She looked both curious and relieved that no one would find out she had these problems. She was still sitting very close to her mom but was making eye contact and even smiling a little.

We started talking about what her worries were, and I explained that all the kids who see me start by making a list of what they're afraid of. I let her know that she could earn prizes for making the worries go away. She became quiet again; it was hard to talk about her fears.

Her mom jumped in. "Is it okay if I start?" Lily nodded.

Mom started with the list of things we needed to work on:

- Staying in her bed
- Going upstairs at night
- Going to sports without a fuss
- Going to school without a fuss
- Doing homework without a fuss
- Taking tests without a fuss the night before
- Not seeking reassurance, since she has the "What if's" about a lot of things (for example, she randomly said things like, "What if I touched the floor and then put my finger in my mouth—could I die?")

I reiterated to Lily that I see lots of kids who have the same problems. Realizing that she was not alone helped her feel less ashamed and more engaged in the process.

We then listed her anxious thoughts:

- For staying in her bed, she said, "I worry about a bad guy coming into my room."

- For going upstairs at night, she said, "I worry there's someone up there."
- For going to her sports, she had to think, but then said, "I worry that I will mess up, and everyone will be mad at me, and when my stomach hurts, I worry I will get sick."
- For school, she said, "I just keep thinking I hate school, and I don't want to go. I know I don't really hate school, but in the morning that's what I think. I just want to stay home and not have to go, and I get really angry about having to go to school."
- For the test anxiety, she said, "I worry I'll fail the test, and I worry the teacher will get mad at me."
- For her other random worries, she said, "I just worry I could do something that could make me sick or die."

As her parents listened, I could see they were surprised at how strong her fears were. Her father moved toward her and kissed her forehead. He understood more how hard this was for his little girl.

Then we forged ahead.

Step 2: Rate the Anxious Behavior

We went through the list again, and Lily rated how hard she thought it would be to work on these symptoms. She rated them on a scale of 0 to 10, with 0 being easy and 10 being impossible:

- Staying in her bed she immediately said was a 10. She started to cry and say, "I can't do it! I get too scared." I quickly explained to her that we would break it down so she could accomplish this in steps. The first step would be for her to try to stay in her bed. If she went into her parents' room, her dad would bring her back to her bed but stay there in her room until she fell back asleep. She looked relieved and said, "I think that would be about a 7. Okay, I guess I could do that, maybe." She didn't sound too convincing. Of course, both parents would have to be on board and ready to do this. I recommended that they think about it and perhaps start when there was a long weekend, so getting sleep was not such an issue.
- Next was going upstairs at night. Again Lily said that was a 10. We discussed breaking it down. We agreed that it would be a 6 if she went upstairs at night but one of her parents was in the room at the bottom of the stairs, and she just went up to get something and then came right down.
- Next was going to her games and practices without a struggle. She seemed

to think that was a 3, although her parents looked surprised at such a low rating. She also rated going to school and doing homework and taking tests with a similarly low rating. She was perhaps overconfident in her ability to control her anxiety. We also knew she was very ashamed of this behavior and confused by it. We discussed how sometimes, when you rate things in my office, it might be different when you actually try to do it; it could be a higher or a lower number. Lily said, "No, I think it really is a 3. I can do it."

• Having her birthday party she rated as a 4. Her parents were surprised that she so worried about this. Her dad said, "Lily, what's the big deal about having a party?" She then looked sad and became very quiet. She said, "I just don't want a party." I reminded them that worries don't make sense, and lots of kids worry about things that they don't need to worry about. Birthday parties can create anxiety for some kids. Lily worried about her friendships, and she worried that her friends wouldn't come to the party, or if they came, maybe they wouldn't have a good time. She couldn't decide if she wanted a party or what kind of party to have. Making these decisions felt overwhelming for her. So the solution was to avoid the whole party thing altogether.

Now it was time to move on to specific goals and get to work.

Step 3: Agree on Challenges to Work On

Lily agreed to try to go upstairs at night, with at least one of her parents staying in the room at the bottom of the stairs. She also agreed to try to control her meltdowns when she was anxious about school and sports. But she didn't want to work on staying in her bed.

Her dad's immediate reaction was "This is not an option, Lily. You have to do this." He clearly was frustrated by this sleep situation.

She then started crying again and said, "I can't do it!" Her anxiety in even talking about it was all over her face. She even started shaking.

This goal seemed too hard for her right then, and if we pushed her to do something she was not ready to do, we could cause this whole plan to fail. If the goal is too high, kids often shut down, feeling they can't do it. They then can become angry and resistant. We knew this was Lily's pattern. She also needed a sense of control because her anxiety could make her feel so out of control. So we needed to respect her limits at this point, to get her to agree to do this work. Lily needed to gain more confidence in her ability to manage her anxiety, and then she would be more ready to tackle sleeping independently.

So, it was agreed. Dad had to wait until Lily was ready to work on her sleeping. Dad was not happy, but he reluctantly supported the plan.

Next was the birthday party. At first Lily insisted that she just didn't want a party. Her mom and dad felt that this was strange since she went to parties and had lots of friends. The anxiety this caused her was confusing for them. Lily didn't want to recognize that this was anxiety related but said, "Okay, if it means that much to you, I'll have the party." Her birthday was in four weeks, so that was a timely goal.

Now, we needed to move from goals to strategies.

Step 4: Initiate and Teach Strategies to Practice

Lily needed to understand how to challenge her anxious thoughts. This is the cognitive part of the therapy. We talked about how to label these thoughts and see them as something to observe, without reacting to them, and not to believe anxious thoughts are true. We discussed what to label them; she thought for a few minutes, and then said, "fake fears." Okay, we would call her worries fake fears. This was her label that she thought of. She needed to think of these thoughts as lies in her head that she would not believe.

Her biggest fear was that an intruder would come into the house. She knew that was not realistic, yet when she had these thoughts, she became very frightened.

Her dad reminded her that their dog barks at flies that come into the house, never mind a stranger. Lily laughed, which was wonderful because anxious kids need to learn to laugh at their irrational worries and not be so serious. Laughing puts the worries in perspective.

Then he added, "On our block the biggest intruder has been that skunk we've all smelled."

Now she was really laughing. Humor works beautifully to take the power out of anxious thoughts, when the anxious person is not currently flooded with fear. When Lily was not experiencing anxiety, that was the time to help her begin to change the way she thought about her worries.

Eventually, she needed to realize that these thoughts were "fake fears."

Our goal was to help her take the power out of the thoughts. She could learn to label them and practice putting her attention on what was important, in the here and now. This mindfulness would allow her to accept these thoughts as irrational and let them go. She could then focus on soothing, calm, happy thoughts or on the activities she was engaged in.

We discussed how this practice would help her at bedtime. Music or an audiobook helps a lot of kids relax at night. Even though she clearly stated that she was not ready to work on sleeping alone, the seed was planted for her to know strategies that could help her, when she was ready.

Since she agreed to work on no fussing before school, sports, or tests, we needed to discuss strategies to help her. She needed to review her anxious thoughts and have "replacement thoughts." These are thoughts that are based on reality, not her fears.

For all her worries about the "bad guy," we discussed what she could say to herself to "talk back" to the anxiety. "I am safe in my room and in my home. My parents are here, and they take care of me. These are my fake fears, and I don't need to pay any attention to them."

For her school anxious thoughts, she said, "I don't love school, but it's okay. I'm smart, and I have friends who like me. Recess is always fun."

For her fears before tests, she said, "I'm a smart girl. I studied, and I will do the best I can. If I get things wrong, no one will be mad at me. It's okay; I don't have to be perfect." I also encouraged her to write down her worries before a test. Writing down the specific worries helps kids make them concrete and more able to let them go, instead of going into the test with this vague dark cloud of nervousness over their heads.

For sports, Lily said, "I'm a good player. I am getting better, and no one's perfect. I don't have to be perfect. I always have fun when I play, and I will have fun."

As we were discussing these thoughts, her mother was writing the replacement thoughts down, so Lily could read them when she was feeling anxious. That was an excellent strategy to help Lily stay focused on what's real, and not on her irrational thoughts, when she starts to get anxious.

Lily also agreed to have a "calm-down list," which included things that she could use to calm herself down when she started to worry.

Lily's Calm-Down List:

- She agreed to make a special playlist on her iPod of her favorite happy songs to listen to.
- She likes the feeling of playing with silly putty.
- She's a good artist and enjoys drawing pictures of animals.
- She loves to write stories about mermaids.
- She always feels happy riding her bike.
- She likes to play basketball and focus on getting the ball in the hoop.
- She loves to sing and dance by herself in her room in daylight.

We discussed how she needed to use this list. When she noticed she was getting anxious and upset, she needed to try to calm herself down. If her parents noticed, they could prompt her to calm herself down. I reminded her parents that they can't calm Lily; she needed to learn to calm herself. Lily and her parents were getting the message that Lily had to take control of her emotions. Her parents could support her, but she needed to do the work.

The work continued with practice.

Step 5: Note and Chart Progress Made

Lily and her parents agreed on how to chart her progress. They decided to record the date, what she worked on, the difficulty rating, and how many points she earned. Her parents figured out how many points she could earn and what the points were worth.

Lily agreed and was excited, but she wondered what the points meant. This led us to the "perks."

Step 6: Offer Incentives to Motivate

We now discussed what she could cash in her points for—what rewards she wanted to earn. Right away, Lily said, "I want a new puppy!" This family already had a dog. A pet is often what kids want for a prize, but it's not a good reward, unless the family has already agreed on it. Mom and Dad had clearly said no more pets. So we had to move on.

Lily was deflated for a few minutes, but we quickly started coming up with other ideas. I reminded her that prizes didn't have to be things; they could be experiences.

So we made a list of rewards she could earn points for:

- Breakfast with Dad   **30 points**
- Picking the restaurant the next time her family goes out to dinner **20 points**
- Extra 20 minutes on the iPad **20 points**
- Miniature golf   **30 points**
- Picking a movie to watch **25 points**

- Sleepover with two friends (her parents hate sleepovers!) **75 points**
- Getting a manicure with Mom **40 points**
- Going on a hike with Dad, without brother   **15 points**

She was now very excited about earning her points and receiving prizes.

Step 7: Reinforce Progress and Increase Challenges

After two weeks, we met again.

Lily was thrilled to tell me her progress. She had struggled at first with going to sports without a fuss. It was harder than she thought, but she was having success. She was proud to show me her chart and how her numbers had gone down.

She showed me her latest ratings for all the goals she'd been working on:

- Going upstairs. This was now a 0! She proudly told me she was not scared anymore as long as Mom or Dad was in the room at the bottom of the stairs when she went up. We discussed increasing that goal, with Mom or Dad able to be anywhere in the house when she went upstairs. She agreed and said that would probably start out at a 5 rating of anxiety.
- Mornings with no fuss. This had been going very well. Most of the time she did it, but on some days, she lost it and melted down, crying and screaming. We discussed what had happened on those days. Usually the meltdowns were triggered by something not going smoothly in the morning, including fighting with her brother, having a hard time picking what to wear, or not being hungry for breakfast. We discussed how to use music in the morning to help her keep calm. We also discussed again how to talk

back to her anxious feelings. She still wanted to work on this, so it stayed on her chart.

- No fussing with sports. This was something she had been mastering. She now said it was about a 3 and much easier. She'd been reading her positive thoughts before getting in the car and enjoying music in the car. Now she said she didn't have to read the positive thoughts—she remembered them—but would continue to use music. This also stayed on her chart.

- Fussing before tests. This was also much better. She had a big standardized test coming up soon, so we decided to keep this on the chart until she got through that test. We identified her anxious thoughts about the test, and she would write them down.

- Birthday party. She had planned for her birthday party and was looking forward to it. It was in less than a week. We discussed how, right before the party, she might get worried and might need to use her calm-down list to help her. She had to remember to challenge her anxious thoughts. She could now get points for working on staying calm before the party and not having a meltdown. Her parents now understood, in advance, what could trigger her anxiety and were learning to help her be prepared with strategies that would help avoid difficulties.

Overall, Lily had done a great job meeting these challenges and seemed very happy with herself. But we still had to address her hardest goal: sleeping in her bed, something she hadn't been able to do for years. She looked upset and didn't want to talk about it. We discussed breaking it down, with the first step being a parent sitting next to her bed until she falls asleep. I reassured her that they would not leave until after she was asleep. Lily said she would like to listen to a book instead of music at night. We agreed it should be a book she'd already read, so she wasn't staying up to hear what came next—distracting but not stimulating. Her mother or father would stay with her, but after they said goodnight, the lights would go out, and the book would go on.

At that point, there would be no more talking. It would be as if the parents were not in the room. I made it clear that if Lily tried to talk to her mom or dad after this point, they would ignore her. It was time to go to sleep. She agreed to start with that.

Once Lily was comfortable with this approach, which would probably take several days, her parents would then move their chair closer to the door but do the same routine. When she was comfortable with that, they would move the chair out of the room, step by step, until she could fall asleep alone in her room.

Lily was reminded that her fears at night were "fake fears," and that she needed to label them and focus on the book she was listening to. We discussed the points, and I suggested she get 10 points for the first night she does every new step, and 5 points for practicing the same step until she was comfortable. She agreed and was excited to earn so many points.

We discussed when she would start this. A long holiday weekend coming up seemed ideal, because no one had to get up early for school or work, so there would be less anxiety about getting sleep. We all agreed that she would start then, and we talked about one new prize she wanted to earn, another audiobook. Lily's dad had never looked happier. He was eager to sleep in his bed instead of on the couch.

In short, while Lily continued to make progress, getting through all the steps was a process. She was learning that she was the "boss" of her brain and that she could control her worries. That is always a breakthrough.

Next Steps

Lily continued to make progress with her worries. After a few weeks of working on sleeping in her own bed, she was sleeping independently through the night. Her parents were thrilled. They didn't realize it could be changed so quickly. They've learned how to anticipate Lily's triggers for her worries and help her in advance to use her strategies to relax and stay in control. Now, Lily continues to earn prizes, and things are much better. They don't need to meet together anymore but agreed that if things get difficult again, they will come back for a "tune-up."

Dagan and Sheila's Story

GAD affects kids of all ages. Eric is a teenage example. His parents met with me first.

His father, Dagan, started: "We are here because of our 16-year-old son. Eric's a great student, a star soccer player, who plays year round, and a terrific kid. The problem is, he worries way too much. He worries not only about getting into college, but the other night, he was worrying about never finding a good job after college, and not having enough money to live . . . For god's sake, he's 16 years old! He worries about other things too. He's always studying like crazy before a test, and then he can't sleep because he worries he won't get a good enough grade. He stays up to all hours of the night doing homework. His grades, by the way, are fine. He tells us he always has trouble sleeping, because, I guess, there's always something this kid can worry about. I don't get it. He has a great life, and what does he have to worry about, really?"

Sheila then added, "What really has us concerned is that he's a great athlete, but he worries that he doesn't have strong enough muscles. I know teenage girls worry about their bodies, but I didn't know boys did. He wants to get a six pack, and he worries that he's fat. He's not fat. He works out in the gym and plays soccer all the time, and he's in great shape. For the last couple of months, he's been worrying about food. Out of the blue, he doesn't want to eat this or that, because it has too much fat or too many calories. I don't want him to start getting some crazy eating disorder on top of everything else. He still eats his ice cream and French fries, but he has a lot of worries about it."

Sheila wondered about the differences between their children. "He has an older sister, and we never had these problems with her. Are boys different with puberty? Do you think he could have other worries about his body? He needs help to stop worrying so much and to enjoy these teenage years."

Dagan added, "He also is a bit of a hypochondriac. I mean, any little ache or pain or minor illness, he blows way out of proportion. He worries he has a tumor or some horrible disease and is going to die. We have to keep telling him he's fine. And Sheila and I are in good health, but I swear, we even sneeze and he's all over us with questions about what's wrong with us. He worries we are going to get sick and die. He's done this since he was a little kid."

When I asked about family history, both Dagan and Sheila were very open.

"I'll be honest with you," Dagan said. "My brother died of a heroin overdose. Eric doesn't know the whole story. He thinks it was a heart attack. It happened seven years ago, and Eric was so young, we didn't want him to get all worried and upset. My brother used to be a worrier, just like Eric, but then he got into drugs, and there was no helping him. God knows we tried. He was in and out of treatment centers. My poor parents, what they went through with him . . . I tell my kids, whatever you do, stay away from drugs. I think this whole legalizing marijuana is a big mistake."

Sheila interrupted. "Dagan, let's not get into that now. Tell her about your cousins."

"Oh yeah, my cousins, three of them actually, were all diagnosed with ADHD. They were a wild bunch, and one of my sisters, she told me she takes medicine for anxiety, but I thought that was just because of my brother's death. His death really shook us all up. I don't want my kids getting into any of that. It really scares me about Eric."

Sheila then talked about her family. "Well, I certainly am an anxious person. It got really bad after Eric was born. Something about having two kids and the responsibility of it all freaked me out. Then I started worrying that I was going to hurt the baby. It was terrible, and I couldn't sleep. They said it was postpartum depression, but I think it was my anxiety getting out of control. So I started taking medicine, and I still take it. It helps me not to get so worried all the time. My father was a big-time worrier too.

"Mr. Worst Case Scenario. If there was something that could go wrong, he had already worried about it. He was always convinced that the worst thing possible was going to happen. My poor dad, he was always wound tight." Her eyes filled up. "I'm sorry. He just passed away last year, and I still miss him. That was hard for Eric. He was close to his grandfather. I think his anxiety got worse after that."

Dagan agreed. "Yes, that was tough for all of us. He was a great man. Eric became more of a health nut after his death. He was constantly worrying that he might die or we could die. Remember that? He couldn't stop talking about death and dying and how scared he was."

Sheila nodded. "He's better with that now, but you're right. It took months for him to tone down all his worries about death. I guess that isn't normal."

"I have to ask this," Dagan said to me. "Could all this worrying lead Eric into drugs and alcohol? My brother's death killed my parents. They have never been the same. I still feel so haunted by it, wondering if there was something I could've done to help my brother. I couldn't bear to lose my son that way."

I explained to Dagan and Sheila that having an untreated anxiety disorder does increase the risk for substance abuse because it can become a way to self-medicate to reduce anxiety.

Dagan immediately looked worried. We discussed how alcohol and drugs can be relaxing and make the worries, for some kids, go away temporarily, but then they have more problems. On the other hand, I have treated many anxious kids who are afraid of alcohol and drugs because they can't bear to lose control. I had recently worked with a teen who had ended up in the emergency room after smoking marijuana because the feeling of being out of control had caused him to panic, and then he had thought he was dying.

I emphasized that it's important for Eric to learn how to manage his anxiety so he doesn't experience difficulties later. I also suggested that they tell Eric the real story about his uncle's death. Better he hear the facts from them than from someone else, and it might motivate him to stay away from drugs because they took the life of his uncle. With the family history of addiction, he's at higher risk and needs to be very careful about drugs and alcohol. They agreed to tell him.

Okay, Eric was up next.

Eric's Story

Eric wanted to meet alone with me to talk about his concerns.

"I worry about everything. I can't help it. I love soccer, and I really want to get a soccer scholarship. I want to play in college, so of course, in every game I worry about a zillion things. Getting goals, obviously, but then I worry about getting injured. Can you imagine? One big injury, and that's the end of my days as a soccer player. I'm one of the best players on the team, so that has me worried. I feel like, lately, I've been holding back in the field. If I mess up . . . I can't mess up. Even my coach said something about it. He said, 'Keep your head in the game, Eric. What's going on with you? Get out there and score!' Now I'm worried about the coach being upset with me. So much pressure."

He added, "I worry about tests, grades, getting into the right college, getting a job after college. I know I take longer than anyone else doing my homework. I can never feel like I've done enough. How much is enough? What does 'doing my best' mean? Most nights I'm up way past midnight working. When I'm not working on my schoolwork, I feel guilty and worried, thinking I need to work harder."

The worries go on. "I'm starting to worry more about getting fat. I should be in better shape and . . . this is embarrassing, but I worry I'm not developed enough down there, that girls won't like me or guys will laugh at me in the locker room. There's a girl I like in science class, but I'm afraid to ask her out. I keep looking in the mirror, and I don't like what I see. I think I'm fat, and I know I'm not big enough. I can't stop thinking about this.

"I get good grades, although lately it's been harder and harder to keep them up. I have lots of friends, if only I didn't worry so much. I'm tired of it. It's exhausting, and I wish I was like everybody else. Even my friend Rob said, 'Eric, loosen up. What's wrong with you?' I know this can't be normal."

Like most kids with anxiety, Eric thought he was the only one who had these feelings. I let him know that lots of kids share these worries, and we could work on freeing him from worrying so much. After I explained to Eric how cognitive behavioral therapy works, he was eager to begin.

Step 1: Target Anxious Thoughts and Behaviors

We explored Eric's anxious thoughts and behaviors. They generally fell into two categories: the first was worrying and ruminating over various issues. The second was perfectionism, which included worrying about his performance in school and sports. His perfectionism led to working too hard on homework, to the point where he often got fewer than five hours of sleep at night. Most of Eric's anxiety involved thoughts and not behaviors. It was fueled by how he put so much pressure on himself at school, in sports, and with friends, especially girls.

Eric started making his list of anxious thoughts:

- My homework is not good enough.
- I'm going to fail the next test.
- I'm going to stink in soccer.
- I'm not going to have a good life (job, family, money, etc.).
- I'm not strong enough or big enough, and I'm fat.
- I have a fatal disease.
- My parents have a fatal disease and will die.

He also listed his anxious behaviors:

- Overproducing on my homework and spending too much time making it perfect.
- Studying much more than is needed for tests.
- Becoming more restrictive in my eating, due to worries about getting fat.
- Examining myself in the mirror to make sure I'm not getting fat.
- Checking the size of my penis and researching penis size on the Internet.
- Seeking reassurance from my parents.

At this point, I needed to explore whether Eric was depressed in addition to his anxiety. Depression is a serious illness that affects many teens. When I asked him about his mood, he denied any depression. He said he can get down about the worrying, but if he didn't have all those worries, he'd be fine. Significant anxiety can be depressing, a normal reaction to anxiety, not an additional diagnosis. Eric had great friends, a supportive family, and a general optimism about his future.

A thorough assessment of depression is always important to do. After assessing Eric, I felt confident that he was not suffering from any mood disorder but was experiencing the saddening effects of his anxiety disorder. I also screened him for suicide risk, which is critical to do with every patient. Sometimes parents are afraid to bring up suicide for fear that it might give their child this idea. To the contrary, openly asking about suicidal thoughts is crucial. Eric was clear that he had no suicidal thoughts or other thoughts about wanting to hurt himself. He just wanted relief from his anxiety.

"Most of the time, I'm pretty happy," he said. "I'm just exhausted from worrying so much. I wish I could make it stop."

I told him we were on the right track.

Step 2: Rate the Anxious Behavior

We talked about how Eric had to change the way he thinks as well as some of his behaviors. We discussed how hard it would be to make these changes. Eric then rated the difficulty on a scale of 0 (easy) to 10 (impossible).

- Not worry about college and his future **8**
- Not worry about soccer **6**
- Be more aggressive in soccer and not hold back **3**
- Not worry about tests **8**
- Set limits with homework **8**
- Not worry about girls **5**
- Ask a girl out **4**
- Not worry about his body **4**
- Not examine his body in the mirror **5**
- Not seek reassurance about his body **8**
- Not be picky about his food **3**
- Not seek reassurance about the fat content of food **2**
- Not worry about having a serious illness **4**
- Not seek reassurance about a serious disease when he is not feeling well **7**
- Not worry about his parents being so sick they will die **3**
- Not seek reassurance from his parents when they are sick **4**

Step 3: Agree on Challenges to Work On

Eric looked seriously at his list for what seemed like a long time. He couldn't decide what to work on. He was demonstrating for me how he tends to overthink everything and become overwhelmed. He then seemed to get lost and unfocused on what he needed to do. He needed to be reminded that there was no perfect choice. I suggested he break it down by focusing on the easiest first. It was clear how tasks could take him a long time because he got very caught up in the details and couldn't see the whole picture. I had to remind him that this choice didn't have to be perfect; he should just pick.

Once I helped him break it down, he agreed to the following:

- Be more aggressive in soccer.
- Stop being picky about his food.
- Not examine his body in the mirror.
- Not seek reassurance about his body or food.
- Ask a girl out.

The goals felt challenging but not too overwhelming, so he was willing to start with these and then work up to the harder goals.

Step 4: Initiate and Teach Strategies to Practice

Eric identified his thoughts about soccer. He said, "When I'm playing, and even before the game, I start thinking, *What if I mess up in front of everyone? I will be letting my team down, the coach will be disappointed, and no one will think I'm such a good player anymore. I won't get a scholarship, I won't go to college, and I will have a terrible life.* Once I start thinking this way, I get more afraid to even try to score."

We then discussed what the realistic thoughts are:

- I'm a good player. I work hard at developing my skills, I want to score, and no one's a perfect soccer player.
- If I mess up, everyone will not be focusing on that, and it won't change the way they think of me.
- My coach likes me and has confidence in me.
- My team needs me to put myself in the game and play the best I can.
- If I don't get a scholarship, I can still go to college.

He then identified his anxious thoughts about food:

- If I eat this, I will get fat.
- If I get fat, girls won't like me.

Next, we worked on replacement thoughts:

- I don't have a weight problem.
- I'm a healthy eater.
- Everything is fine in moderation, and I enjoy food.

Then he listed his anxious thoughts about his body:

- I'm getting fat.
- I don't have enough muscles.
- Girls won't like my body because I don't look strong enough, and my penis is too small.

Replacement thoughts:

- I'm healthy and fit; there is nothing wrong with how I look and how strong I am.
- I'm not too small, and my penis is normal. My doctor told me everything about my body is normal.

Eric revealed that there's a girl, Lucy, in his science class that he's friendly with and wants to ask out but has been too afraid.

His anxious thoughts are:

- What if she says no? I'll be humiliated.
- I don't know how to ask her.
- I can't think of where to go with her.
- What if she really doesn't like me?

Replacement thoughts:

- She's always friendly and seems to like me.
- I could text her and ask her if she wants to go to the movies this weekend.
- If she says no, I tried, and it doesn't have to be such a big deal.

We discussed his seeking reassurance. He agreed to stop it and, when he gets the urge, to remind himself that it's just his anxiety and he doesn't need to focus on it. He then agreed to read these lists of anxious thoughts and replacement thoughts every day to help him keep focused on what is rational.

Eric seems to have a lot of free-floating anxiety. "I feel like I'm always stressed, and I can't relax."

We discussed the use of mindfulness in managing his anxiety. He agreed to work on meditation, using a meditation app on his phone, for fifteen minutes a day. I also talked with him about observing his anxious thoughts but not engaging with them—keeping a distance from them. Labeling them helps with this, as does realizing that these anxious thoughts are meaningless and not important. Keeping his focus on the here and now, what is really going on around and within him, will help him relax.

Next, we discussed other relaxing activities he could build into his life. He already exercised, which was helpful. We talked about using music, which he loves. He agreed to listen to music before bed as a way of relaxing and turning off his worries. He needed to get more sleep, but he was still very driven to work too much on homework. That was something he needed to work on, so he agreed to practice these strategies to help manage his stress and to proceed with our steps.

Step 5: Note and Chart Progress Made

Like most teenagers, Eric had his phone with him all the time, so keeping track of his work on his phone made the most sense. In the notes section of his phone, he listed his anxious thoughts and replacement thoughts. He put in a daily reminder to review them.

Before each soccer game, he would write concrete goals for himself, and after the game, he would review how well he did with them. For example, he decided to take a shot at a goal anytime the ball was near and he had a chance, instead of avoiding it.

He thought afternoons, after school, would be the ideal time for him to take fifteen minutes to meditate. He put reminders in for that.

He also made a playlist to listen to at night to help him relax before bed.

Step 6: Offer Incentives to Motivate

Eric felt that he did not need incentives, but he wanted his parents to know what he was working on. We invited them to join us toward the end of the session to learn about his goals. Eric shared that he was going to really make an effort at not seeking reassurance from them. They were very supportive and asked if they could do anything to help. Eric suggested that if he forgot and asked for reassurance, they could remind him that his anxiety was talking and not answer his anxious questions. Dagan then asked what they should say to Eric if he asks for reassurance. Eric thought for a few minutes and then said, "Just say 'Stop.'" They agreed.

Step 7: Reinforce Progress and Increase Challenges

After three weeks, Eric was happy to report his progress. He had gone to the movies with Lucy. He had been much more engaged in soccer, and his coach had recently commented on how his game had improved. He had worked on not seeking reassurance about food and his body, and his worries about both were much lessened.

Eric had been applying the music and meditation strategy, but not every day. He complained that his life was so busy, it was hard to find time. He said that even with the reminders, he would be busy doing something else, and then forget. He reported that his school worries had gotten worse, and he was still getting very little sleep. Math was particularly difficult, and his grades were falling. He was getting worried about taking the SAT, even though it was six months away. He said, "I can't stop thinking about college and getting into a good school and worrying I won't be able to. I'm getting more and more stressed. All my friends are starting to talk about college, and that's really making me crazy."

We invited his parents into the conversation. They agreed that he'd made good progress with the things he'd worked on, but they were seeing him get less sleep and worry more and more about school.

Sheila said, "He got a C on his last math test, and I thought it was going to put him over the edge. He's never gotten a C before, and he's working so hard. We don't know what to do to help him."

We discussed several options. One was to consider a medication evaluation. Another was to consider having a neuropsychological battery of tests done to see if there might be something, other than anxiety, that could be making it harder for him to reduce his time on homework. He might have organizational or attention difficulties, or an undiagnosed learning disability. Once we had more information, the skills and strategies to help him would be clearer.

Eric and his family decided to get the testing and postpone discussion of medication. He agreed to keep working at the CBT as well, since there had definitely been progress.

Next Steps

Eric got the results from his neuropsychological evaluation and it showed that, in addition to anxiety, he had attention deficit hyperactivity disorder (ADHD), which was contributing to his academic difficulties. He was a smart kid, so the ADHD had not been a problem until he encountered the increased demands of high school. In the earlier grades, he was able to do well even without paying attention. High school was different. If he got distracted, he quickly fell behind. Falling behind triggered his anxiety, which distracted him more. This had become a vicious circle for Eric and was a major reason his homework took so long.

Anxiety disorders and ADHD often go together, and each one makes the other worse. An anxious child who is distracted and unable to concentrate and know what is going on becomes more anxious. An impulsive child who blurts out answers or interrupts others becomes more anxious due to feeling so out of control. In addition, anxiety can be distracting; sitting in class and worrying about things can make it difficult to concentrate. Anxiety can also make some kids appear hyperactive. Noticing if the symptoms of inattention and hyperactivity are still present when a child is not anxious can give a clue as to whether these are symptoms of generalized anxiety or of two separate conditions. It is important to tease this out, and sometimes that's best done through a comprehensive neuropsychological evaluation, which is what helped Eric and his parents understand his challenges.

The combination of a neuropsychological evaluation and the clinical information about anxiety can be useful in sorting out the cause of a child's distraction level. Many kids have both ADHD and anxiety, and on the surface, the symptoms can look the same, but asking key questions helps figure out what is causing the distraction. A common example is parents complaining about the long showers their kids are taking. With ADHD, the long showers are caused by kids standing in the shower spaced out, relaxing, and not realizing how the time is passing. Kids with anxiety are in the shower for a long time worrying that they might not be clean enough and feeling they need to wash more and more. On the surface, the symptom is the same: forty-five-minute showers. But the cause is very different. The same dynamic is seen with a child who is distracted in school. Is the child daydreaming or busy worrying? It looks the same to the teacher, since the child is not paying attention, but the cause is either lack of attention, intense worrying, or, as in Eric's case, both.

Eric had a difficult time maintaining attention and then would panic when he realized he had missed what he needed to be doing in school. The more anxious he was, the more difficult it was for him to pay attention. His ADHD fueled his anxiety, and his anxiety fueled his ADHD. Both needed to be addressed. He is now working with a tutor to help him stay organized, and his parents have requested accommodations at school, including extra time for tests and being able to sit in the front of the class so he has fewer distractions.

Eric also had a medication evaluation and has been taking medication for his anxiety and to improve his attention. Eric and his parents report much progress, and they have a greater understanding about what has made things so difficult. His grades have improved, he's getting more sleep, and he is worrying less. He tells me that it's easier to use the strategies we discussed, and he can more easily push away the worries. His parents report the most important thing for them: Eric seems much happier.

Eric is a good example of how complicated kids can be. Because he has always had high anxiety, it was easy to assume that anxiety was his only problem. Yet his ADHD was greatly contributing to his anxiety. Understanding this helped us work on all the issues he was struggling with, not just his anxiety.

DSM-5 Guidelines

The *DSM-5* identifies the diagnostic criteria necessary for a diagnosis. The assumption is that many readers will have children who meet some but not all the criteria.

Generalized Anxiety Disorder

A. Excessive anxiety and worry (apprehensive expectation), occurring more days than not for at least 6 months, about a number of events or activities (such as work or school performance).

B. The individual finds it difficult to control the worry.

C. The anxiety and worry are associated with three (or more) of the following six symptoms (with at least some symptoms having been present for more days than not for the past 6 months):

Note: Only one item is required in children.

1. Restlessness or feeling keyed up or on edge.

2. Being easily fatigued.

3. Difficulty concentrating or mind going blank.

4. Irritability.

5. Muscle tension.

6. Sleep disturbance (difficulty falling or staying asleep, or restless, unsatisfying sleep).

D. The anxiety, worry, or physical symptoms cause clinically significant distress or impairment in social, occupational, or other important areas of functioning.

E. The disturbance is not attributable to the physiological effects of a substance (e.g., a drug of abuse, a medication) or another medical condition (e.g., hyperthyroidism).

F. The disturbance is not better explained by another mental disorder (e.g., anxiety or worry about having panic attacks in panic disorder, negative evaluation in social anxiety disorder [social phobia], contamination or other obsessions in obsessive-compulsive disorder, separation from attachment figures in separation anxiety disorder, reminders of traumatic events in post-traumatic stress disorder, gaining weight in anorexia nervosa, physical complaints in somatic symptom disorder, perceived appearance flaws in body dysmorphic disorder, having a serious illness in illness anxiety disorder, or the content of delusional beliefs in schizophrenia or delusional disorder).

American Psychiatric Association. "Generalized Anxiety Disorder." In *Diagnostic and Statistical Manual of Mental Disorders*. 5th ed. Washington, DC: American Psychiatric Association, 2013.

Attention-Deficit/Hyperactivity Disorder

A. A persistent pattern of inattention and/or hyperactivity-impulsivity that interferes with functioning or development, as characterized by (1) and/or (2):

1. **Inattention:** Six (or more) of the following symptoms have persisted for at least six months to a degree that is inconsistent with developmental level and that negatively impacts directly on social and academic/occupational activities.

   Note: The symptoms are not solely a manifestation of oppositional behavior, defiance, hostility, or failure to understand tasks or instructions. For older adolescents and adults (age 17 or older), at least five symptoms are required.

   a. Often fails to give close attention to details or makes careless mistakes in schoolwork, at work, or during other activities (e.g., overlooks or misses details, work is inaccurate).

   b. Often has difficulty sustaining attention in tasks or play activities (e.g., has difficulty remaining focused during lectures, conversations, or lengthy reading).

   c. Often does not seem to listen when spoken to directly (e.g., mind seems elsewhere, even in the absence of any obvious distraction).

   d. Often does not follow through on instructions and fails to finish schoolwork, chores, or duties in the workplace (e.g., starts tasks but quickly loses focus and is easily sidetracked).

e. Often has difficulty organizing tasks and activities (e.g., difficulty managing sequential tasks; difficulty keeping materials and belongings in order; messy, disorganized work; has poor time management; fails to meet deadlines).

f. Often avoids, dislikes, or is reluctant to engage in tasks that require sustained mental effort (e.g., schoolwork or homework; for older adolescents and adults, preparing reports, completing forms, reviewing lengthy papers).

g. Often loses things necessary for tasks or activities (e.g., school materials, pencils, books, tools, wallets, keys, paperwork, eyeglasses, mobile telephones).

h. Is often easily distracted by extraneous stimuli (for older adolescents and adults, may include unrelated thoughts).

i. Is often forgetful in daily activities (e.g., doing chores, running errands; for older adolescents and adults, returning calls, paying bills, keeping appointments).

2. **Hyperactivity and impulsivity:** Six (or more) of the following symptoms have persisted for at least six months to a degree that is inconsistent with developmental level and that negatively impacts directly on social and academic/occupational activities:

Note: The symptoms are not solely a manifestation of oppositional behavior, defiance, hostility, or a failure to understand tasks or instructions. For older adolescents and adults (age 17 and older), at least five symptoms are required.

a. Often fidgets with or taps hands or feet or squirms in seat.

b. Often leaves seat in situations when remaining seated is expected (e.g., leaves his or her place in the classroom, in the office or other workplace, or in other situations that require remaining in place).

c. Often runs about or climbs in situations where it is inappropriate. (**Note:** In adolescents or adults, may be limited to feeling restless.)

d. Often unable to play or engage in leisure activities quietly.

e. Is often "on the go" acting as if "driven by a motor" (e.g., is unable to be or uncomfortable being still for extended time, as in restaurants, meetings; may be experienced by others as being restless or difficult to keep up with).

f. Often talks excessively.

g. Often blurts out an answer before a question has been completed (e.g., completes people's sentences; cannot wait for turn in conversation).

h. Often has difficulty waiting his or her turn (e.g., while waiting in line).

i. Often interrupts or intrudes on others (e.g., butts into conversations, games, or activities; may start using other people's things without asking or receiving permission; for adolescents and adults, may intrude into or take over what others are doing).

B. Several inattentive or hyperactive-impulsive symptoms were present prior to age 12 years.

C. Several inattentive or hyperactive-impulsive symptoms are present in two or more settings (e.g., at home, school, or work; with friends or relatives; in other activities).

D. There is clear evidence that the symptoms interfere with, or reduce the quality of social, academic, or occupational functioning.

E. The symptoms do not occur exclusively during the course of schizophrenia or another psychotic disorder and are not better explained by another mental disorder (e.g., mood disorder, anxiety disorder, dissociative disorder, personality disorder, substance intoxication or withdrawal).

American Psychiatric Association. "Attention-Deficit/Hyperactivity Disorder." In *Diagnostic and Statistical Manual of Mental Disorders*. 5th ed. Washington, DC: American Psychiatric Association, 2013.

Chapter 4

Silent Liza and Hidden Patrick

Selective Mutism and Social Anxiety

Selective mutism is an anxiety-based disorder in which the anxiety is focused on speaking. It is an extreme form of social anxiety, which is why these disorders are grouped together in this chapter.

Selective Mutism

Children with selective mutism usually speak freely and normally at home but are mute in other situations, particularly at school. The disorder is often evident when they go to preschool and do not speak at all. Their anxiety can be so severe that they are often described as having the "deer in the headlight" look of sheer terror when expected to speak. There are many myths about these children, including that they have been traumatized or that they are just stubborn, with overprotective mothers. Nothing could be further from the truth. Selectively mute children all have one thing in common: anxiety.

With a phobia about speaking, children with selective mutism often don't want any attention from others. Birthday parties with singing and a cake can feel overwhelming, and eye contact can be difficult when others are speaking to them. At the same time, most of these children, to the surprise of others, are chatty and outgoing at home with their immediate family.

Early intervention with these children is crucial. The longer this disorder goes on untreated, the harder it is to treat. Teenagers with selective mutism have already lived silent lives. They get by; schools often make accommodations for them, enabling their silence. They frequently have no friends, because it is hard to be a nonverbal friend. Silent play dates may work in preschool, but not in adolescence. They have become the child who doesn't speak, and staying in that environment makes it difficult to speak. If they are known as the child who doesn't speak, they think that to start speaking would draw attention to them. These kids hate that attention; it increases their anxiety. Ironically, selectively mute kids who are placed in a different environment, among people who don't know they don't speak, will often have an easier time speaking.

Selectively mute teens may seem odd because they have not had normal social development. Their lives are limited yet all too comfortable because of the well-meaning accommodations given to them. Motivating these older children with selective mutism becomes very difficult. At that point, parents are desperate; many have tried traditional therapy or medications, which have failed. They worry about how their child can ever become independent. These teens are not easy to treat, because they are so used to getting by without speaking.

Unfortunately, I have seen far too many of these teens, which motivates me to advocate strongly for early intervention with selectively mute kids. Many of these older kids who have been selectively mute for many years often have an additional diagnosis of being on the autism spectrum. They often speak fully at home, however, without any language difficulties.

In the following pages, you will hear one family's story about their daughter's selective mutism and how they used the TRAINOR Method to change behaviors. The TRAINOR Method focuses the cognitive behavioral therapy on training parents to apply CBT strategies to help their child speak in social and school environments, without focusing on getting the child to speak with the therapist. The idea is that spending a lot of time getting children to speak with the therapist does not easily translate to the children speaking where they really need to speak, to their friends and in school. Focusing the intervention specifically on the child's environment, with parents and teachers working together to directly apply CBT strategies, is a more effective and powerful approach to curing selective mutism.

Isabella's Story

Isabella came to me because her daughter, Liza, was in kindergarten and not speaking. At our first visit, this is how she described the situation: "Liza is 5—smart, funny, and a delight to be around. We have a 3-year-old daughter, Ariel, and our son, Patrick, is 7. Liza plays well with her brother and sister, and honestly, if you saw her running around our house screaming and laughing with her brother and sister, you would think nothing's wrong." Isabella began enthusiastically, but then she turned serious. "Obviously something is very wrong. She doesn't speak at all in school, not even to her teacher. She doesn't talk to the other children, although she plays with them, and they like her, and she gets invited to all their birthday parties. Liza talks at home when she gets ready for school, but her silence begins when I walk her to the bus stop. As soon as we get close, she becomes silent, even though her best friend is there."

Isabella sighed, then continued. "Her problem with speaking is not just in school. She doesn't speak to some of her aunts and uncles. She speaks to my mother, but not much to my father. My husband's parents live out of state, and when they come to visit, she's quiet at first but then warms up to them and talks. In restaurants, she talks freely to us but usually asks us to order her food." I was beginning to get a picture of Liza, and the family's dynamics, as Isabella went on to share more.

"Her best friend, Annie, is in her class and lives on our street. They play together almost every day. She talks to Annie when she comes to play at our house, and she is normal with her when she plays at Annie's house, but she doesn't speak to Annie's parents. And at the bus stop and school, she doesn't even speak to Annie, which must be confusing for her." I asked Isabella how long this had been going on.

"I first realized this was a problem in preschool," she said. "I spoke to her pediatrician, and he said I should 'leave it alone' and she would 'grow out of it.' Now she's in kindergarten. She's not growing out of it. If anything, it may be getting worse." Isabella took a deep breath, then slowly exhaled. "I worry because other people never get to see the real Liza—the bubbly, chatty girl we know. They see this silent girl. Liza can already read, but her teachers don't know that because she's so silent at school. She's smarter than they realize. She likes school and is happy to go," Isabella explained. "But when she comes home, she talks and talks and is really hyper and can be mean to her younger sister. I wonder if it's because she's been so silent at school all day."

At this point, I asked Isabella what Liza had told her about her silence. "When I try to talk to her about talking, she gets angry and won't discuss it. I've tried ignoring it, and I've tried getting angry about it. Nothing works. Frankly, when she doesn't answer people who talk to her, she looks rude. I usually answer for her and say something about her being shy. I feel embarrassed. I don't know what to do to help her." Then Isabella introduced information about her husband. "Her father tries, too," she said, looking away a moment, then back at me. "He jokes about it with Liza, and tells me to lighten up about it. He had anxiety as a child, so he's more tolerant than I am. I find myself getting so annoyed, feeling like those two are buddies and I'm the bad guy." Here, Isabella stopped and leaned her head in her hand. "I'm very worried about her."

The parents' story, of course, is from their perspective. When the child finally feels safe talking to someone about it, her story begins to unravel the mystery.

Liza's Story

Having worked with many hundreds of kids with selective mutism, I know Liza's story. I know it from what these children tell their parents, and I know it from what they tell me when they are cured. I am very practical in my approach to working with these children. My goal is not to get them to speak to me; it is to get them to speak in their world. I could spend many hours weekly to get them to speak to me, but that would be limited to once or twice a week, and I need them to be talking to people in their daily life, which doesn't include me. Focusing my therapy on getting them to speak to me seems a waste, since it will not generalize to others. Even when these kids are very comfortable, they often still communicate nonverbally. The TRAINOR Method places the focus on helping selectively mute children to speak by working with their parents. Their parents, whom they love, want to please, and are most comfortable speaking to, hold the key to their recovery. Parents can be the bridge to them speaking to other important people in their lives. My role is to guide their parents. This is Liza's story, which I have learned through working with many selectively mute children and their parents.

"I hate when Mommy and Daddy talk to me about talking. I hate it when they ask why I don't talk. I hate when they tell me to talk when we go places. I can't and I won't! It feels too bad. I don't know why it feels bad to talk. I guess I just don't want to feel those bad feelings. It's easier to not talk. Why do I have to talk? Maybe I'll talk when I go to first grade or when I'm six. I just want everyone to leave me alone about this. It's too hard."

Liza was a smart little girl, and like most selectively mute children, she had no specific answer to "Why don't you talk?" This often perplexes adults, who believe there has to be a reason. The reason is anxiety. Most of us can remember anxious moments when we were younger, or even as adults. Remember how bad anxiety feels? Hot and red in the face, shaking, scared, heart beating, trouble breathing? That is how Liza felt when asked to talk. She truly did not know why. She just knew she didn't get those bad feelings when she didn't talk, so silence seemed the way to go.

Her parents knew better. They knew that talking was not optional, and they worried about the future if she did not get over this. Once I explained that cognitive behavioral therapy (CBT) would help change the way Liza thought about talking and help change her speaking behavior, they knew they wanted this treatment for her.

But first, I met with Liza's parents, without Liza present, for several good reasons, including those I have mentioned but want to emphasize:

- Liza hated people talking about her talking. It made her feel embarrassed and angry.
- I was a stranger to her. Why would she want a stranger to know about this?
- Liza needed help talking in her world of school and teachers, peers and relatives. More important than her talking to me was my guiding the family to help her talk in places where it would make a difference in her life.
- Most important, Liza spoke freely to her parents. They were a link between her talking world and her silent world. They needed guidance to help her break through this anxiety. Working with Liza's parents and helping them apply the TRAINOR Method was the most effective approach to help Liza.

Step 1: Target Anxious Thoughts and Behaviors

First, we had to identify the thoughts that supported her anxiety. Remember, we look for thoughts that support the common defenses of denial and avoidance. For Liza, these thoughts included the usual denial—"I don't have to talk"—and avoidance—"It feels bad to talk and good to not talk, so I'm not talking." Her parents heard this reasoning from her all the time.

Liza's parents quickly learned that it was important for them to have a consistent and firm message to Liza that challenged her denial and avoidance and, at the same time, normalized her struggle. They learned to tell her things like "All children must talk, and you will also talk. You just need help to talk. It's not an option to not talk. Talking is hard for you, just like riding a bike is hard for some kids (you're great at that!), and with practice, you will talk like all the other kids. You're not shy; you just need help with talking." This message was firm and supportive, exactly the tone her parents needed to use to help her overcome her phobia of speaking.

Liza's parents made a list of all the situations where Liza did not talk and all the people in her life she did not talk to. When it came to talking, how was Liza different from other kids her age? Here is their list:

Liza does not talk

- at school
- at gymnastics, swimming lessons, or any summer camps she has attended
- at the bus stop
- to people who talk to her when shopping with her parents
- to her aunt Beverly or uncle Jim
- to Aunt Cindy
- to Uncle Peter
- to her doctor or dentist

Liza does talk

- at home with her family members
- with Annie at Annie's house and at Liza's house

- on other play dates at her house
- in restaurants, most of the time
- to her grandparents
- to her siblings' friends when they are at her house

Step 2: Rate the Anxious Behavior

Liza's parents talked to her about how difficult it would be for her to talk in these different situations. She, of course, did not want to talk about it, but her parents encouraged her, introducing the prizes she could earn by cooperating.

Since she was so young, we kept the rating system simple: Easy; Hard; Very Hard; Very, Very Hard. Here are her ratings:

Talking:

- at school
  Very, Very Hard
- at lessons and camp
  Very, Very Hard
- at the bus stop   **Hard**

- to people who talk to
  her when shopping   **Very Hard**
- to her aunts and uncles   **Hard**
- to order her food in
  restaurants   **Easy**

Step 3: Agree on Challenges to Work On

Liza's parents had a good idea of how hard all these speaking challenges would be for her—very, very hard. We discussed breaking the challenges down to be more manageable.

Talking at school was a big priority, so we listed several options:

- Liza talking to her parents as they get closer to the bus stop
- Mom taking Annie and Liza away from the large group of kids at the bus stop and playing a quick game with them where they have to talk, such as a guessing game
- Having more play dates at her house with the children from her class so that they hear her voice, and she experiences herself talking to them
- Having one of her parents play with Liza and Annie in the classroom after school so that she can experience herself talking in the classroom

- Once Liza has mastered talking in the empty classroom with her friend, introducing the teacher gradually into the room, so the teacher hears Liza's voice while she is playing

This list was a start to help Liza become desensitized, step by step, to talking. Because Liza talked freely with her parents, we hoped that they could introduce this list to her when she felt relaxed at home.

Liza's parents left my office with the challenging task of talking to her about these goals and getting her agreement on what to work on first. They needed her to buy into this plan, because she had to do the work of practicing these steps. I reminded Liza's parents to reinforce her speaking behavior and give her incentives for any time she speaks in a way she never spoke before. She needs to get the message that the more she speaks, the more she gains. She has a phobia of speaking. It makes her extremely anxious, and she would like to simply stay silent. As a little girl, she doesn't understand why this is not a choice she can make. She needs a lot of encouragement and a strong consistent message from her parents:

- She can do this.
- It will get easier as soon as she talks.
- Worrying about talking is a "silly worry"—we laugh at those worries and push ahead.

Since Liza is a little girl, we decided to call the steps a "talking game," so she would want to play. I reminded her parents to be firm, supportive, and positive. Liza felt scared, like she could not talk in difficult circumstances; they could help her by making sure the goals were challenging but not overwhelming. By keeping a positive "You can do it" attitude, Liza's parents could help her learn to talk back to the fear and push herself past it. She could learn to "just do it!"

Liza agreed to talk to her parents as they neared the bus stop. She also agreed to work on having more play dates with two girls from her class, Keesha and Jamie. And she would play with Annie after school in her classroom with her father present, when no one else was there. This was a great list of starting goals.

Step 4: Identify and Teach Strategies to Practice

The cognitive strategies involved reinforcing the same message to Liza: "You can talk. All kids must talk. You will talk, and we will help you. You can do this. It will get easy for you." The message also included the idea that she's not shy. Some selectively mute children get the idea that it's okay not to talk because they are shy. Liza's temperament was not quiet. At home, without anxiety, she was a chatterbox who wanted to be an actress. She needed to learn that her anxiety about speaking was something she had to push through. The behavioral strategies involved doing this step by step. Liza learned that she needed to push herself to do it—"Don't think about it, just do it!"

Step 5: Note and Chart Progress Made

I encouraged Liza's parents to make a "talking chart" of her speaking challenges and have her color and decorate it. Even at 5 years old, she needed to take charge of this process because she needed to do the work. Her chart listed the goals she had agreed to and had spaces for bonus stickers. Her parents explained to her that she could earn bonus stickers if she did any "new" talking behavior. Her parents said they would carefully notice when she spoke in a situation where she had not talked before, and later, they would reward her with a bonus sticker. This gave her the message that every time she fought her fear of talking, she won at the talking game. Her talking chart was done. It looked pretty, all decorated by Liza. She felt excited, but we all realized that fighting her fear of speaking would be hard work for little Liza.

Step 6: Offer Incentives to Motivate

We asked Liza to work hard at fighting her anxiety. She started with the attitude that she liked her pretty chart but didn't want to do this and really saw no reason she should. She was not motivated to work at this talking game. Incentives would motivate her. Liza knew that her parents were getting a big prize box with presents for her to pick from every time she did a new speaking behavior. In the prize box were coupons for special time with Mom or Dad, craft items she enjoyed, puzzles, books, and hair bows—all things she loved.

By playing this talking game, she would win stickers and prizes. Every new speaking behavior meant a prize. Practicing that behavior earned her a sticker, and three stickers won another prize. The first time she talked with Annie at the bus stop, she would earn a prize. After practicing it three more times, she would earn three stickers and another prize. With practice, talking to Annie at the bus stop would be natural.

What first felt uncomfortable quickly became easy. Once something on the list is easy, it is crossed off with much praise, and the next challenge is worked on. Step by step, Liza learned that fighting her anxiety is difficult at first, but that it quickly gets easy and feels good.

As part of this process, everyone helping Liza with her talking needed to remember several things. First, when she talked, no one should react. No praise for her. Liza would be anxious in that moment and would not want any attention on her. Teachers and others needed to act as though she had always talked like this. That would reinforce for her that talking is no big deal—she could do it! Later that day, long after her talking accomplishment, she would get her prize and praise, and she would feel happy and proud. Not praising is counterintuitive for most teachers and parents. Teachers are so eager to praise a child who makes progress. For children with this disorder, however, it is their nightmare that people will make a fuss about their speaking and draw attention to it. So everyone has to act like speaking has no importance. Then after, when the child is home, praise and incentives can be offered and readily accepted. In addition to rewarding Liza for reaching her goals on her list, whenever she did a new talking behavior that was not on her list, she would earn a prize.

For example, when Liza talked to a child at the playground, her mother noticed that was something she had never done before. It was not on Liza's list, but when they returned home, she received a bonus prize. She knew that the next time she talked at the playground, she would get a sticker; three stickers equaled another prize. Her parents paid close attention to the prize process, which reinforced Liza's speaking progress. She learned that the more she spoke, the more prizes she would get, and the easier speaking would become.

Step 7: Reinforce Progress and Increase Challenges

I continued to meet and guide Liza's parents every few weeks as they helped Liza talk more and more. Once a talking behavior became easy, we raised the goal. Liza's teacher was in daily communication with Liza's parents, reporting on progress at school so she could get her prize and stickers when she came home. Daily feedback was essential because quick reinforcement was important for Liza. If she was not rewarded until Friday for something she had done Monday, she would not even remember doing it.

Liza worked hard, and it took time, but she learned to push herself. She and her parents eventually added another anxiety-producing behavior—using the bathroom at school. Many selectively mute children do not feel comfortable using the school bathroom, even when they can nonverbally ask to go. Since first grade would mean full days at school, her parents felt concerned about this. The first step Liza agreed to was to go to the bathroom after school with her mother and then work up to using it during school. Liza's progress with pushing herself when fearful built on itself. She talked more and more, earning her prizes; gradually she became cured of selective mutism.

Some children with selective mutism simply have a phobia of speaking, just as some adults with minimal anxiety have a single irrational phobia—for instance, flying or snakes. These selectively mute children tend to be popular in preschool, even though they don't speak. I have worked with children like this who show no other signs of anxiety once they overcome their selective mutism, including one child who went on to speak on national TV!

Other children with selective mutism also have additional symptoms of anxiety, including perfectionism, separation anxiety, or obsessive compulsive symptoms. These children may need to manage different symptoms of anxiety in the future. The strategies they are learning to overcome their selective mutism will be useful for other anxiety issues, include recognizing the anxiety, setting goals, and not letting anxious feelings cause them to withdraw and avoid challenges.

Next Steps

Liza continued to make progress and even had breakthroughs. She seemed to make baby steps and then, when she was ready, big steps.

She was increasingly talking to her peers and her teachers. Her teachers learned to create opportunities for her without pushing her. They supported her being engaged with peers she liked but didn't put pressure on her to speak. Knowing she would get rewarded at home helped Liza push herself. Her teachers learned to give daily feedback to Liza's parents about her talking progress, but not to give Liza any praise in the moment. This was hard for them, because they clearly saw her progress and instinctively wanted to praise her. They learned that paying attention to Liza as she moved into the talking world would only cause her more anxiety. Together Liza, her parents, and her teachers were very pleased with her continued progress.

Social Anxiety

Social anxiety is one of the most difficult forms of anxiety to identify and to work on, especially when it is not very severe. Parents often don't notice it at first. They have a child who "likes" to stay home and "doesn't like" to do extracurricular activities, play dates, or other social activities. These children avoid as much social interaction with their peers as they can. They often feel more comfortable with younger children or adults. Peer interactions are more anxiety producing. These kids are not on the autism spectrum; their main problem is anxiety.

According to the fifth edition of the *Diagnostic and Statistical Manual of Mental Disorders* (*DSM-5*), kids on the autism spectrum have difficulties using communication for social purposes, struggle with changing communication to match the needs of the listener, find rules of conversation difficult, and can be very literal in their understanding. They experience these difficulties even when relaxed in the context of familiar situations.

On the other hand, children with social anxiety display none of these difficulties when they are in a relaxed setting. By avoiding social opportunities, however, they are missing out on experiences needed for social development and may appear less mature than their peers. Girls I have worked with who have social anxiety are often very attached to their mothers and to the TV. Boys are usually more involved with computer games, and their only social outlet may be playing games.

Here is one young man's story of how he used the TRAINOR steps to work on his social anxiety. Patrick was 13, and his parents, Lori and David, felt concerned because he did not seem to have many friends and spent most of his free time playing video games.

Lori and David's Story

The first day Lori and David came to see me, Lori told me that they'd had Patrick tested because she had started to worry that he might be depressed, have a learning disability, or have social problems. They had searched for answers for more than a year, trying to figure out how to help him. She said that the testing had shown that he was bright and should be doing better at school. It also said he had anxiety. The neuropsychologist who did the testing recommended that he get cognitive behavioral therapy (CBT), which led his parents to me. "That is why we're here," she said. "Can you work with him?" So I asked them to tell me about Patrick.

"Patrick is a great kid," Lori began. "Maybe we're wrong to worry, but he is home alone so much, it doesn't seem right. He's a decent student. I mean, he's no star student, but he passes all his classes. We always thought he was a really smart kid, but in the last couple of years, his grades have dropped. Instead of getting A's, he now gets B's and even some C's. We know he's capable of more. He seems happy, but it just doesn't seem normal for a 13-year-old boy to have no friends."

She paused, then continued. "We tried talking to his school counselor about this, but she said he seems fine, is always with other boys, and there's no problem. No problem? He comes home every day, does his homework, and then goes on the computer to play video games. He barely stops for dinner and then goes back to playing games until bedtime. The phone never rings. He never gets invited anywhere with friends. We never hear about any friends. Weekends he plays video games by himself or tries to get us to entertain him."

Lori hesitated, looked briefly at her husband, and went on. "David gets angry with him and tells him to get off those darn games and go outside. But that doesn't work. David sometimes has no patience with him. I feel sorry for Patrick; it must be lonely for him. He used to have friends when he was little; in fact, he was rather popular."

David spoke up. "I do get angry at him, and I know I shouldn't, but sometimes I think maybe he's just lazy and needs a kick in the pants. That testing said he has anxiety. Frankly, I'm confused. Watching him at home, he seems pretty relaxed, happy as a clam in front of that computer, playing games, drinking soda, and eating chips. Anxiety? I just don't see it. I suffered from anxiety, had panic attacks as a kid. I know anxiety. Patrick doesn't seem nervous about anything. Stubborn, yes. Spoiled, maybe, but I don't see him as nervous at all. I think the kid just may be lazy."

David's view clearly upset Lori. "This is where we disagree. You think he's lazy, but there has to be more to it than that. Patrick has never been a kid to do much outside of the home. He went through just about every sport. We would sign him up, and after a few practices, he would say he hated it and quit. He doesn't like sports, I guess. Then we thought music. We got him piano lessons, but as soon as someone mentioned a recital, he begged us to quit. We even told him he didn't have to do the recital. We couldn't get him to change his mind. No more music lessons. He says he hates music. We can't force him to do things he doesn't like. Frankly, I dread the summer. He refuses to go to camp. Says he hates camp. I imagine him at home, alone, all summer playing those games. He's gained ten pounds over the last six months, and he's starting to look chubby. I worry about that, too. This isn't normal. We need to help him."

Patrick's Story

Patrick came in to meet with me, and he was clearly angry, no, furious, about being in my office. I found out later that he had exploded at his parents when they'd told him about this appointment and had told them he would not say a word to me. Of course, I understand that even meeting with me challenges his denial, and he doesn't want to move an inch out of his comfort zone. The stronger the resistance, the stronger the anxiety. His anger did not silence him, however; he told me quite a lot. I am sure he was hoping he could convince me to tell his parents to leave him alone.

"I don't know why my parents make a big deal about this. I wish they'd just leave me alone. I like playing video games, and I'm good at them. What my parents don't get is that I play with my friends. We play together. They always want me to do more things. I've tried playing sports. I don't like it. It feels awful. And music lessons? No way. I would hate to have anyone listen to me play. I'm not good at it. My parents keep asking me to have friends over. I would never want to invite a kid over. I wouldn't know what to do. What if he hated it and had a bad time? What if I asked someone and the answer was no? I would feel like a real idiot. And I really don't want to go to someone else's house. It would feel so weird. No thanks. I'm most happy at home, playing my games. My dad explodes at me once in a while about being on the computer too much, but I just ignore him and play my games and he forgets about it. My mom yells at me about eating too much, but hey, I get hungry playing. Can't you just tell them to leave me alone? I don't need to see a doctor. I'm fine. The problem is they keep taking me to doctors.

"I also dread teacher conferences. My parents always come home and grill me about why I don't talk more in class. 'Raise your hand more. Your teachers want to hear what you have to say.' Yeah, right. I would probably say the wrong thing, and everyone would laugh at me and think I was a real dork. I'm happy staying quiet. They also get on me about my grades. I do okay. I wish they would leave me alone. I don't want to be the smartest kid in the class, and I'm not in any trouble at school. I do fine."

By the time he was done, I knew that Patrick didn't want my help. From his point of view, he felt no distress. In fact, just the opposite: he felt quite comfortable living his life the way he did. Meeting with Patrick—unless I wanted to play video games with him—would be a dead end. He didn't think there was a problem. He didn't feel anxious—just the opposite. He felt relaxed eating chips and playing video games.

Patrick's parents, however, felt worried, frustrated, and at times, angry and disappointed in Patrick. Mostly they felt helpless and at a loss for how to help him. In addition to having him tested for learning disabilities and ADHD, they read about Asperger syndrome and thought maybe he had that, or maybe he was depressed. I reviewed the testing, and it showed Patrick to be a happy boy, very bright, with social anxiety. In fact, he seemed to have all the classic symptoms of social anxiety. His primary defense against his anxiety was denial and avoidance. He didn't feel anxious because he avoided all situations that would cause anxiety. He participated in no extracurricular activities and said he hated them.

I have never known a kid with social anxiety to say, "I don't want to play soccer because it makes me feel scared and uncomfortable." They feel scared and uncomfortable and decide they hate soccer and quit. This confuses parents because they understandably think they should not force their children to do an activity they don't like. When they don't like *most* things, however, it is a clue that the anxiety is talking. And you never want anxiety to be making choices for your child.

A need for motivation was the biggest issue here. He was a smart kid whose world was growing smaller and smaller because of his anxiety. He experienced strong denial ("I'm happy at home; what's the problem?") and avoidance ("I don't like doing those activities"). Kids like Patrick will often avoid all activities that involve social interaction and performance.

I had already determined that meeting alone with Patrick would get me nowhere fast. I also knew that meeting with Patrick and his parents would be a disaster. His parents would bring up their concerns: "You have no friends, you play too many video games, you don't work hard enough in school, you eat too much junk food, and you're getting fat." Patrick would feel angry and criticized and swear he would never come to therapy again. And if I happened to mention that perhaps there should be some limits on his computer usage, well, I would just become the enemy in Patrick's eyes: "That doctor is an idiot—what does she know? We're not going back there. Are we, Mom? Please tell me we'll never go back there. She's so mean. Please. I'm fine. I don't need any help."

In that scenario, Patrick's parents would likely feel defeated once again and would not want to drag him back kicking and screaming. Understandably, many therapists might also say that if he didn't want help, therapy would not work. Given the way Patrick had set things up, he wouldn't want help any time soon.

So, I met with his parents. They held more power than they realized. They needed validation that, yes, their parental instincts were right. They had reason to be concerned about Patrick, even though his school thought he was fine, and even though he believed there was no problem. (I tend to think parents know best.)

Kids with social anxiety live in smaller and smaller worlds, and because they are in many ways high functioning, with so many strengths, they are at high risk for depression due to their social isolation. Patrick could complete high school longing for friends but feeling excluded. Or he could find other "outsiders" to hang with who might have deeper problems than his. He was also at risk for substance abuse, because most substances feel really good to anxious kids. In addition, he was at great risk for underperforming because he would not compete and take risks, even though he was very smart. He earned low grades despite his ability, and his grades were hurt by his lack of participation. He was involved in no extracurricular activities because he avoided social challenges. This smart, talented guy barely looked average. He seemed "okay" because he drew no attention to himself and was not a problem at school. He got by. In fact, if he had been the smartest in the class, that might have drawn attention and made him feel uncomfortable. Being an average student helped him blend in, unnoticed. This is how anxiety, in a subtle way, leads to underperformance.

His parents needed to understand that Patrick was a kid. He would choose what felt comfortable, not what was best for him. Knowing what is best for him is his parents' job.

Unlimited time on the computer is not healthy. Patrick could not regulate himself. The more computer time he had, the more he wanted. This felt good; doing anything else felt bad. As long as the choice included staying home and playing video games, he would stay home and play video games. Anxiety made these choices for him—deny and avoid.

Step 1: Target the Anxious Thoughts and Behaviors

Patrick did not have thoughts related to anxiety because he denied there was a problem and avoided situations that would make him feel uncomfortable. So the thoughts that needed to be challenged involved his denial, and the behaviors that needed to be targeted included his avoidance.

The first step was a tough one. His parents needed to set limits with video games. I advised them not to associate this with the therapy or we would lose any possibility of his cooperating with a behavioral program. I often recommend parents set these limits around natural transitions: "It's spring/summer/winter/fall/back to school/end of school/vacation/end of vacation, and we need to change the rules about being on screens." His parents needed to assert themselves and set the limit.

Most experts agree that the daily maximum for all screens for kids should be two hours during the week and three hours on weekends. Screens include TV, computers, and phones. That meant a major lifestyle change for Patrick. Both Lori and David had to agree on a limit they felt they could follow through with. Patrick would not be happy with this, so they needed to be ready for a fight and ready to follow through. They discussed it and agreed on three hours during the week and four on the weekends to start. They had the tough job of enforcing this, so their agreement was crucial.

Before we get to how that tough change went, let's look some more at Patrick.

Patrick believed it was okay to avoid situations that felt uncomfortable. This had to change. Summer was coming; it could not be an option for him to stay home alone with no plans and no supervision on his screen time. He needed to become active and connected with other kids his age. Isolation would only strengthen his anxiety. Choosing the right activity for Patrick was important. He could not, for example, be thrown into a baseball camp when he did not know how to play. It had to be an activity where he could feel fairly comfortable with his skills. He would have a high level of anxiety entering a situation like this if he also had to worry about not knowing what to do or not being good at the activity. He would feel completely overwhelmed. Remember, these kids fear embarrassment, failing, and being made fun of by other kids. He needed to enter a situation that was a good match for him.

Patrick's parents mentioned that he was a strong swimmer. A swim team would help him get exercise and be with kids his age. That seemed like a great match for him. Swimming is a comfortable sport for many anxious kids because they just get in the water and it's pretty clear what they have to do—swim to the other side. It is a team sport but a noncontact sport, with clear, predictable expectations.

Now the hard part—motivation. Patrick would not want to do this. He wanted to stay home all summer, play video games, and eat ice cream. His parents needed to be firm and supportive. Targeting his anxious thoughts and behaviors meant that staying home doing nothing could not be an option.

Step 2: Rate the Anxious Behavior

Patrick didn't acknowledge anxiety, but his anxiety became evident, in the form of oppositional behavior, when his parents spoke with him about doing an activity over the summer. He protested loud and clear. Keep in mind that anger is often fueled by anxiety, and this is what was happening with Patrick. So his parents needed to make it clear that he had choices, and his choices helped rate his anxiety. Swim team was one choice, attending a local summer camp another, and being a counselor in training at a camp for much younger kids another. He was not interested in the camp options, so they could be considered too high on his anxiety scale. He considered the swim team to be the least of all evils but still very difficult. He knew a boy on the swim team, so that helped. He still insisted that he was doing nothing all summer, but his parents clearly heard what would be possible for him this summer and what was too hard. His parents knew then that the swim team was a place to start, even though he insisted he was not doing it.

Step 3: Agree on Challenges to Work On

Joining a swim team seemed overwhelming to Patrick, who continued to say he wanted to just sit home all summer, but his parents held their ground. When a goal is too difficult, break it down. How could we make this easier for him? One way was to arrange for him to meet the swim team instructor. Or maybe he needed to take swim lessons to boost his confidence. Another option was to watch the team practice. We broke it down into steps he could agree to. Even though he didn't yet understand that process was about anxiety, his parents knew that as his comfort level increased, he would be ready for the next step. This was not easy for his parents; they needed a lot of support because Patrick kept fighting, convinced his parents would give in to him. The more his parents understood that this struggle was so strong due to his anxiety, the more they realized how important it was not to give in. He needed them to be strong and firm.

Step 4: Identify and Teach Strategies to Practice

At this point, it became important to discuss what made this so difficult for him. Meeting with me made more sense. His parents reminded him that I was someone who worked with lots of kids who struggle with doing things outside the house. They normalized his experience and meeting with me as much as possible. They presented me as more of a coach than a doctor for "crazy weird" kids. Patrick would not want to feel different or weird.

We suggested that Patrick choose whether he wanted to meet alone with me or with his parents. He chose to meet with me alone. At first he complained about the summer plan and even blamed me, so I told him about other smart, "normal" kids I have worked with. I shared with him what some of their feelings were and how they were able to push past them and ultimately feel better about doing more things outside the house. Their feelings had included being embarrassed, feeling like everyone would be looking at them and making fun of them, being afraid of messing up, and so on. I spoke about how they were able to challenge those feelings and replace them with more realistic thoughts. He listened, but I did not ask him to acknowledge that he had any of those feelings.

I confirmed that this was work and not easy. We then moved on to talk about incentives and rewards, and what he wanted to earn by doing this work. I told him that his parents had agreed to work out incentives and rewards with him. When we discussed what he might get out of all this, it brightened his mood. Of course, his parents would have to agree to his wish list.

Step 5: Note and Chart Progress Made

Because of Patrick's resistance to doing this work, emphasizing his rewards, plus negotiating what he was willing to do to get started, was crucial. His initial list of goals included making a chart. It also included coming to therapy to work on his anxiety. In addition, he agreed to meet with the swim instructor. His chart was small to start, with a strong emphasis on rewards, but it was a start.

Step 6: Offer Incentives to Motivate

Motivation is the most difficult aspect of helping kids with social anxiety. We were asking Patrick to move out of his comfort zone and feel uncomfortable feelings. We knew that as he did these things, they would become more comfortable, and he would experience great benefits. He did not yet know this, however. So incentives became very important. What would motivate Patrick to do this work? You guessed it: more computer time and computer games. Why would we reward his efforts with the very thing we wanted to get him away from? Because that was what would motivate him, ironically, to get away from the computer, get exercise, and connect with other kids. So we set up a system with Patrick: for each step he took, he earned points that he could cash in for more computer time or to use toward games. His parents were concerned that they would be manipulated and that he would take the rewards and then stop working on the issues. I guided them to remember that they were in control, and though money had been spent, they could remove new games or extra time if he did not continue with his steps. I also reassured them that most young people do not manipulate as soon as they start experiencing better feelings about leaving the house.

Step 7: Reinforce Progress and Increase Challenges

We then set up a second chart, listing Patrick's goals and the points rewarded for meeting those goals. When he met with the swim instructor, he received 5 points for that, resulting in four extra hours of screen time or ten dollars toward a game. That may seem like a lot, but the first steps are always the hardest. He now knew that this was not so hard, and he wanted more screen time and games. He was on board and working with us, so we could more fully develop the chart. He was willing to do the steps. Next step was to take swimming lessons. One hour of screen time for each lesson, or three dollars toward a game. Next, he would watch the team practice. One hour of screen time for each time he watched, or three dollars for a game. Next, he would join the swim team for a computer game or six hours of screen time. Once he joined, each practice meant one hour of computer time or three dollars toward a game. The first of everything was the biggest incentive, and then doing it again and again earned him less because it became easier for him. This was all charted with his points. We also included a bonus in his chart: if he joined a social activity, invited a friend over, or went to a friend's house, he earned a game or six hours of screen time.

Patrick was able to continue step by step and meet his goals because he was motivated. His parents did a good job of keeping track of his progress and gave him what he earned. As he reached one goal, he moved up, with goals always increasing.

If it had not worked, we would have had to reevaluate. Are the goals too high? Do we need to break them down into more steps? Are the incentives strong enough? Patrick needed to be motivated to do this work, and his parents had to stay united and firm in setting limits, as well as be supportive in providing him rewards and praise.

As Patrick continued to make progress, his parents were pleased with his reduced anxiety. By the middle of summer, he had experienced success in swimming, participating in the team as well as in team matches, even winning a ribbon now and then. We expected him to build on this. As summer came to an end, we established new goals for the fall, including extracurricular activities, increased class participation, improved grades, and continued swimming on the school's swim team, where he had some friends now. We met regularly together, sometimes all four of us, to negotiate with his parents these new goals and incentives.

Patrick had started to break out of his comfort zone of computer games and chips, but his parents had to learn to understand his anxiety, provide reasonable goals, and support his progress. In this process Patrick was experiencing success, which builds on itself. The swim team was a start, a first of many steps for Patrick.

Next Steps

Patrick continued on his journey. With limits set on his screen time, he was more motivated to do other things, especially with the incentives. His parents learned to pick their battles but to be firm in their expectation that he participate in activities and not withdraw. They also learned to give him the support he needed so that the goals were not too challenging for him.

Kids like Patrick are so anxious about trying new things that they need their skills to be strong. Often that means preparing them before they join a group activity so that they have confidence in their ability. Just signing them up for something they *should* be good at isn't enough; they need to go into the activity with confidence, so they only have to battle their social anxiety. If they have to feel their social anxiety on top of worrying about not doing well and not knowing what to do in an activity, that's far too overwhelming. Patrick's parents understood this, so Patrick was able to feel successful when he did his swimming, and this success led to more confidence, which led to more success.

DSM-5 Guidelines

Social Anxiety Disorder (Social Phobia)

The *DSM-5* identifies the diagnostic criteria necessary for a diagnosis. The assumption is that many readers will have children who meet some but not all the criteria.

A. Marked fear or anxiety about one or more social situations in which the individual is exposed to possible scrutiny by other. Examples include social interactions (e.g., having a conversation, meeting unfamiliar people), being observed (e.g., eating or drinking), and performing in front of others (e.g., giving a speech).

   Note: In children, the anxiety must occur in peer settings and not just during interactions with adults.

B. The individual fears that he or she will act in a way or show anxiety symptoms that will be negatively evaluated (i.e., will be humiliating or embarrassing; will lead to rejection or offend others).

C. The social situations almost always provoke fear or anxiety.

    Note: In children, the fear or anxiety may be expressed by crying, tantrums, freezing, clinging, shrinking, or failing to speak in social situations.

D. The social situations are avoided or endured with intense fear and anxiety.

E. The fear or anxiety is out of proportion to the actual threat posed by the social situation and to the sociocultural context.

F. The fear, anxiety, or avoidance is persistent, typically lasting for 6 months or more.

G. The fear, anxiety, or avoidance causes clinically significant distress or impairment in social, occupational, or other important areas of functioning.

H. The fear, anxiety, or avoidance is not attributable to the physiological effects of a substance (e.g., a drug of abuse, a medication) or another medical condition.

I. The fear, anxiety, or avoidance is not better explained by the symptoms of another mental disorder, such as panic disorder, body dysmorphic disorder, or autism spectrum disorder.

J. If another medical condition (e.g., Parkinson's Disease, obesity, disfigurement from burns or injury) is present, the fear, anxiety, or avoidance is clearly unrelated or excessive.

Specify if:

Performance only: If the fear is restricted to speaking or performance in public.

American Psychiatric Association. "Social Anxiety Disorder (Social Phobia)." In *Diagnostic and Statistical Manual of Mental Disorders*. 5th ed. Washington, DC: American Psychiatric Association, 2013.

Chapter 5

Where Are You, Mom and Dad?

Separation Anxiety

Separation anxiety is both normal and healthy when babies are between 8 and 14 months old. In fact, if babies don't experience both an attachment to their parents and a fear around strangers at that age, it's cause for concern. Sometimes anxiety about being away from parents continues in a milder form for several years. Separation anxiety after the age of 6 years old, however, is a cause for concern.

Children with separation anxiety often become very worried when they're not close to a parent and sometimes also to their home. They often worry something bad will happen to their parents if they're away from them. This may lead them to feel as if each separation could be a final one, which is the cause of a panic reaction. Parents leaving their screaming child with a babysitter will often be frustrated and say, "We're only going to the movies. We'll be back in a little while." But saying that over and over again makes no difference. To the child, clinging and screaming, "Don't go!" it's as if Mommy and Daddy will never come back.

This is another good example of how irrational anxiety is. When in this anxious state, children can't hear what's being said to them. They are in panic mode over what seems to be nothing to their parents. To these children, this feels like the last time they're seeing their mom and dad, so of course they're screaming, "Don't go!"

Some kids with separation anxiety don't worry so much about something bad happening to their parents; they worry that, without their parents, something bad will happen to them. They don't feel safe in the world unless they're close to their parents. Whatever the worry—that something bad will happen to their parents or to them—the anxiety is the same.

They feel most safe and comfortable being close to their parents, often one parent, usually their mother.

Kids with separation anxiety are the kids who have trouble being left at birthday parties, play dates, after-school activities, and, at its worst, school. They want their parents to stay with them, even when all the other kids are glad to have their parents leave. This can feel embarrassing, because now the clinging and screaming is happening in public, with other kids and parents looking on. When kids are flooded with this anxiety, they often don't care who sees them out of control, to their parents' surprise. Again, they're not thinking; they're only feeling overwhelming fear. They are reacting to this intense feeling of danger if their parents don't stay with them.

Separation anxiety disorder can be a small component of generalized anxiety disorder or a part of other anxiety disorders. Sometimes, however, separation anxiety disorder stands alone. Either way, the strategies for reducing this anxiety are the same: the step-by step method of establishing goals to change the thinking and behavior associated with the fear of separating from parents.

Kids with separation anxiety often complain of physical symptoms: stomachaches, headaches, and other pains of unknown origin. Do they really feel the pain caused by their anxiety? Or are they saying they're in pain to avoid the separation? Does physical pain become a more acceptable and effective way of communicating emotional pain? Though we will never know the answer to this, my guess is that it's probably a combination of all of the above. Kids are smart and learn pretty quickly that saying, "I'm scared; I don't want to go" will quickly be dismissed, often with annoyance, by their parents. Saying, "I can't go; my stomach hurts so much—it hurts, it hurts" will not be so easily dismissed. In fact, often the opposite occurs, and it becomes their pass to both stay home and get sympathy. We also know that when severely stressed, people commonly develop stomach pain and a lack of appetite.

Some kids, when anxious, get headaches, which may be in response to the stress. Headaches and stomachaches can be symptoms of anxiety. They can also be an excuse for a child to say, "I can't do this." We will never know how many kids really feel pain and how many use this as an expression of their anxiety. They may be "faking it," but they are doing that for a reason. They feel too overwhelmed by their fears.

Kids with separation anxiety, like other anxious kids, often have a hard time sleeping independently. Sleep often feels like the ultimate separation. They may cry and scream unless a parent stays with them until they go to sleep. They can have what look like panic attacks if they are left alone at night. Often they won't even go to their bed. They have to sleep in their parents' bed. Or if they fall asleep in their bed, with their parent with them, they may then wake up, panic, and run into bed with their parents. This makes sleeping a big issue for the whole family. Parents frequently give in, for many good reasons. They want everyone to get their sleep, including siblings, who could waken if the anxious child starts throwing tantrums in the middle of the night. Everyone has to go to school or work the next morning, and sleeping with Mom and Dad could mean everyone sleeps, albeit at a cost.

When an anxious child is in the parents' bed every night, some parents find themselves being "kicked out" of their bed and end up sleeping on a sofa or in the child's bed. Some parents give up and just put a mattress on the floor next to their bed for their child to sleep on.

Parents can be surprisingly accommodating to kids with separation anxiety. Why? Because it's so much easier than struggling with their child, fighting battles they can't seem to win. These kids, at any age, may throw huge temper tantrums when pushed, and parents naturally learn how to avoid these major struggles, often by enabling the anxiety. When patience is gone, however, parents often react with anger and frustration. A mother of a 12-year-old said, "When she won't go to sleep and keeps coming out of her room, and it's later and later, I am not at my best. I have had it, and I yell at her. I have to get to sleep, and it's just too much. I'm angry, and sometimes I lose it. It is not my best parenting moment, but there's only so much I can take! I give in. We all have to sleep."

Separation anxiety, like all forms of anxiety, can be very difficult to live with, but families like those described below can learn how to help their children manage their anxiety.

Casey and Kenneth's Story

Casey and Kenneth came to get help with their daughter, Kara.

Casey started. "Kara is 7 years old, and a delight. She's a happy little girl, but she's always had trouble leaving me. In preschool they had to peel her off of me, screaming, every morning. The teachers always said that once I left, she was fine. I can't tell you how many times I would be crying in my car as I drove away. It was so hard to see her like that. By the last year of preschool, she seemed fine and able to go to school, no problem. Then came kindergarten, a new school, new kids, new teacher, and it started all over again—the tears every morning and again not wanting me to leave when I dropped her off.

"Every night, getting her to sleep was a battle, with her crying about school. Her teacher was amazing, so nurturing and understanding. She would meet me and quickly whisk Kara into the classroom and get her involved in an activity. She said Kara was fine after that."

She continued. "First grade, the same thing happened, but it only lasted several weeks and then she was okay. This year she's in second grade, and in the beginning of the year, again it was rough, but now she goes to school with no major problem."

Kenneth added, "She really likes school, and she's smart, has lots of friends. She can be shy sometimes, but she's a happy little kid. Sometimes I think my wife's making too big a deal about this. I think she'll outgrow it all if we leave it alone. She's a very normal kid. Casey, you have to agree."

Casey got defensive. "I agree, she's normal most of the time, but it's not normal to need me to go to birthday parties. She's the only kid who can't be dropped off at these things. If I try to leave, she starts crying. And soccer practice, other parents don't have to stay there the whole time. She panics if she thinks I won't be there. The same with everything she does. You don't see it, because you're at work, and she's not the same with you. She always needs me with her, and frankly, it's starting to get embarrassing. None of her friends need their mother or father with them at all these activities. She may outgrow it, but in the meantime, she literally has a panic attack if I try to leave her. That can't be good for her, and that's not normal."

Casey took a breath and continued. "And we both know her sleeping with us isn't right, but we've just gotten used to it. It used to be in our bed, but it was so uncomfortable, we just put a cot next to our bed. So now, our 7-year-old sleeps in a cot next to our bed. This isn't normal. Kara has never been able to sleep independently."

Kenneth interrupted. "That's not true. Remember last year? She slept in her own bed for months."

Casey disagreed. "Yes, but who had to stay with her until she fell asleep? And when she woke up in the middle of the night, almost every night, where did she end up? In our bed. Let's face it, that's not normal behavior for a 7-year-old. Also, she still has temper tantrums like a 2-year-old. It often happens when I need to leave her, but it's ridiculous. She's too old for all of this."

The stage was set for me to meet with Kara and her parents.

Kara's Story

Kara spoke first. "I need my mom to be with me. I don't know why. I worry, 'What if something happens to me and she's not there?' I feel safe with my mom being close. I feel all alone and scared if she's not with me. At school, now it's better, I'm used to it, and I don't feel scared anymore. But birthday parties and soccer and dance, she can't just leave me there all alone. I get scared and need her to stay and not leave. I need her to stay with me.

"At night I can't sleep unless I'm close to my mom and dad. I just get scared. I don't know what I'm afraid of. I just can't do it. I feel cozy and safe when I'm sleeping in my mom and dad's room. Their bedroom is so warm and comfy. My room feels too scary to sleep in. I need to be with them at night."

I encouraged her to continue.

"My mom gets mad at me sometimes because of this. I can't help it. I just need to be with her. When she gets mad, it makes me mad, and it makes me cry more. I just need to be with her. I need it. I don't even want to talk about it. I just want everyone to leave me alone. It's the way

I am, and there's nothing wrong with it. It's not that bad."

Kara is like most anxious kids with separation anxiety. She's healthy in so many ways and seems happy and relaxed until she has to be in a situation without her mother. She doesn't worry that something bad will happen to her parents; she worries that something bad will happen to her, and her parents won't be there. She feels alone and vulnerable without her parents being close, especially at night. Sleep represents a major separation for many kids, and being without Mom and Dad feels very dangerous and scary for Kara.

Also like many anxious kids, Kara wants no part of any therapy that will force her to separate from her mother. She's convinced she can't do it, and she's angry that anyone would try to make her. She wants everything to stay the same, and she's very happy in her comfort zone with her mother and father staying close to her. She sees no need to change and doesn't even want to discuss it. In short, while Kara came to meet with her parents, she made it clear she didn't want to change anything. Talk to her about anything else, however, and she's a cute, charming girl.

Step 1: Target Anxious Thoughts and Behaviors

Kara stressed that she was angry at her parents for talking about her anxiety. I realized that forcing her to participate and asking her to talk about her anxiety would only create more anxiety and more distress and opposition.

Knowing that she needed to feel as comfortable as possible, I asked her parents to draft a list of her anxious thoughts and behaviors. The understanding was that if they got it wrong, she would correct them.

Her mom started with a list of her conception of Kara's thoughts:

- I always need Mom to be with me. (Hearing this, Kara looked up and got defensive. "Not all the time, just sometimes.")
- If something bad happens to me and my mom and dad aren't there, I'll be in danger.
- My room is too scary at night.
- I am only safe at night if I'm with my parents.

Her mom then looked at Kara and said, "I know what you're thinking right now . . . This is not a problem. I don't need to change this, and I can't change this without feeling too scared."

Kara added, "Yes, it's too scary, so why do we even have to be here? I want to go home now. How long do we have to be here? I hate this. I told you I didn't want to come here. Why did you force me? Take me home. I'm leaving!"

Her father then jumped in. "Kara, STOP THIS. We're not going anywhere. The appointment's not over yet."

Kara folded her arms and stared at him but said nothing. She was clearly angry.

Her father looked at me and apologized. "She's not usually like this. She's usually a very polite girl."

I knew that talking about these fears was making her anxious, and when she got anxious, she could quickly become angry. Many anxious kids get angry and oppositional when confronted with their fears. Understanding Kara's mindset, I offered her candy, which I always have in my office. She perked up when I gave her a lollipop. Sucking on the lollipop contained her anxiety for the moment by providing a pleasant distraction.

Next, I wanted to list her anxious behaviors. Kara still refused to talk, so her dad then began listing her anxious behaviors:

- Sleeping in our room
- Having her mom stay with her at birthday parties and all after-school activities
- Crying and not wanting to leave her mom every year when school starts
- Not wanting to go to camp because her mom can't be there
- Needing her mom to go on school field trips with her
- Needing to sit with us at school events instead of sitting with friends

He then reassured Kara. "See, that's not a long list. Just a few things we need to work on. You can do this!"

Kara still did not look happy, but her arms weren't folded anymore.

She picked up one of my toys and started fiddling with it, although she still had no interest in participating.

Optimistic nevertheless, I suggested moving on to the next step.

Step 2: Rate the Anxious Behavior

Kara again wanted no part in this step, but her mother explained to her that she's the only one who knows how hard these things will be.

Slowly, we persuaded her to help us with the rating system:

- Staying at birthday parties without her mom   **10**
- Going on field trips without her mom   **10**
- Sitting with her friends, not her parents, at school events   **10**
- Going to after-school activities without Mom   **10**

- Not crying every year when school starts   **10**
- Going to camp   **10**
  "I'm never going to camp, and you can't make me!"
- Sleeping in her room   **10**
  "I can't do that! Don't even say that to me!"

With Kara rating everything at least a 10, or impossible, we weren't doing very well. To make things worse, not only was Kara angry with us, but her parents were angry with her.

Kenneth was exasperated. "I knew this wasn't going to work. She needs us. I'm sorry, but she's just not ready for this."

Casey then looked annoyed at both Kenneth and Kara. "Who's the boss here anyway?" she said. "This stuff has to change. Kara, you have no choice in this. It's not normal to need me all the time, and your friends are going to start making fun of you and calling you a baby. This isn't 7-year-old behavior. You're too big for this now. Like it or not, you have to change this. I'm not putting up with this anymore." Kara started crying this time, really loudly.

It was apparent how much power this little girl wielded in this family and how her anxiety caused so much conflict. Casey was determined to force Kara to be more independent and was angry because she felt no support. Kenneth and Kara wanted no part in this.

Quickly, the family dynamics unfolded: Dad gives up and wants to avoid conflict with Kara; Mom fights with Kara and threatens her; Kara cries and screams until everyone gives up and feels hopeless.

The root of this was that Kara felt very anxious and was fighting to stay in control. So we were stuck in this cyclical family experience. Anxiety was winning this game, and nothing was about to change. But the good news was that the family dynamics playing out illuminated what life was really like at home. It became clear how stuck they felt and why they needed help.

At this point, I knew the direction had to be changed quickly since everything was moving toward anger and hopelessness. I started asking about what Kara could earn by doing all this work. I also let Kara know that she didn't have to make all these changes right away. We could break it down into steps, little steps for her. I told her I wouldn't force her to do something that was too hard for her. I told her she could be the boss of this work, but that we had to work together.

That reasoning caused her to look up and stop crying. As I considered the approach going forward, I knew she wanted to be in control and was desperately afraid of being forced into feeling those horrible scared feelings. Up until now, it had seemed like there were only two choices: keep everything the same and stay comfortable and close to her parents or be forced to do things she ostensibly couldn't do, that made her feel overwhelmed. Clearly, she needed to be the boss and feel like she had control of her out-of-control anxious feelings.

The more I reinforced that she would be the boss, the more relieved Kara looked. But she was not quite a believer yet.

Casey picked up on Kara's change in attitude and said, "Kara, you can do this, and we'll help you, and you'll earn prizes. Maybe you could earn getting a manicure, or a trip to the arcade with your friends, or getting a frozen yogurt with your dad. And you know what's coming soon? That new movie you want to see. I bet we could take a couple of your friends to see that with you."

Dad smiled and added, "I'll even let you get some candy at the movies." Kara looked surprised, like that was a big deal, and said, "My dad is a health nut and makes us give out raisins for Halloween."

Kara demonstrated how her mood could quickly shift, as with most kids. Once she felt she had regained her control, she could relax, and it was like all that crying had never happened.

Okay! Now we had to talk about the work ahead.

Step 3: Agree on Challenges to Work On

Together we looked at the list of anxious behaviors.

We decided to start with after-school activities, because they happen every week. Practicing challenges makes the activity easier, so frequency is important. Kara didn't have another birthday party to go to for a while, but soccer had two practices a week, and she went to dance once a week.

At all of Kara's activities, her mother couldn't leave; she had to stay right where Kara could see her. I suggested we start with Mom going to the bathroom and coming back. Kara would know this was going to happen—no surprises. Her mom would go to the bathroom, and if Kara saw that her mother wasn't there, she would know that she was coming back in a few minutes.

Casey immediately said, "I never thought of going for just a few minutes. I thought the goal would be I just drop her off."

I asked Kara to rate how hard it would be if her mother left for a few minutes to go to the bathroom or get a drink of water. She thought about it and said, "She's not going to get in her car and leave?"

Her mom reassured her that she would not leave in her car. Kara then said it was a 6. I reminded her that she would earn points for doing this, toward her prizes. We then agreed that her mother would do the same thing during her dance lessons. Kara said that this would also be a 6. I reminded Kara that there would be no tricks, no surprises. If we say that her mom will go to the bathroom, she won't leave instead.

Next, we looked at school field trips. There was one in two weeks to the science museum. Kara immediately got upset and said to her mom, "I need you to come, or else I won't go."

Casey responded, "You have to go. You don't need me there. You can do this. Don't think you're staying home from school because of this silliness."

Kenneth looked away, and Kara started crying. Here we go again. Kara felt like she couldn't do this, Mom was angry and frustrated, and Dad wanted nothing to do with the fighting between the two of them. I reminded them that when this happens, we have to break it down. It seemed like it should be easy, but for Kara, it felt too hard. I suggested that Mom go on the field trip as planned, but not sit with Kara, and that Mom lead a group that Kara wasn't in. So Mom would be there but not close to Kara during the trip. Kara looked relieved and said that would be a 5.

That didn't sound like much of a change to her mother, but Kara needed baby steps to build her confidence. If the goal felt too hard, we were creating a battle that couldn't be won. Kara had to be engaged in this process for it to work. Now we had a plan for the after-school activities and the field trip.

Again, I reminded Kara that she would earn points for all this work. I also reminded Mom and Dad that we had to work together. If we set the goal too high, everything would blow up.

And so the (baby) steps continued with number four.

Step 4: Identify and Teach Strategies to Practice

For this step, we looked at Kara's thoughts. Her primary thought was that she couldn't be alone in these situations without her mother because she thought something bad would happen to her, that she would be in danger. We all spent some time challenging that thought. Kara needed to be actively involved in this discussion. Talking at her would not be effective. She would just tune that out. So we started by asking her what she thought would happen. She didn't know. Like many kids with anxiety, she wasn't necessarily aware of her anxious thoughts. So I suggested we brainstorm. What could happen if Mom was not there?

"I could get sick," Kara said. "The coach could get sick. It could start raining on the soccer field, and we wouldn't be able to practice. I could get hurt at dance. I could get lost at a field trip and not know where to go. Some bad guy could come." Kara admitted that the chance of anything like this happening was very small. But what if it did happen?

I asked Kara to explore each scenario and what she'd do if her mom wasn't there. Her responses:

- If I got hurt at dance or soccer, the teacher or coach would call my mom and she would come.

- If I got sick, I could tell the grownups, and they would help me until my mom came.

- If I got lost on a field trip, I would go to a police officer and ask for help.

- If a bad guy came, I would run to my teacher or my coach and scream for help.

We all reinforced the fact that her parents only leave her in safe places. She was reminded that she was always with responsible adults, whose job it was to take care of her.

Her dad joked, "Kara, you act like we are dropping you off in the middle of a jungle with lions and tigers and bears all by yourself. We're talking about Miss Lucy's Dance Studio and soccer practice with Mr. Williams and Mr. Cooper. They're not lions and tigers and bears." Kara laughed, which is always a good sign.

We then discussed the need to talk back to the anxiety when she gets these fears. She could laugh like she just did, remembering she's not in a jungle. We asked what she could say to herself when she gets anxious. She smiled and said, "I'm safe. I'm not alone with lions, tigers, and bears."

So a little humor led to progress.

Step 5: Note and Chart Progress Made

We then discussed making a chart, which Kara, the artist, wanted to decorate.

- She would earn a point for each after-school activity her mother was able to leave for a few minutes.
- She would earn 5 bonus points if her mother left five times in a row and she was fine.
- She would earn 5 points for going on the field trip and not in a group with her mom.
- She would get 10 bonus points if she stayed away from her mom the whole trip.

I also explained that bonus points could always be awarded if she did something else she hadn't done before that allowed Mom to separate from her. After she did these brave things, she had to rate how hard it was for her on a scale of 0 to 10.

On to the incentives.

Step 6: Offer Incentives to Motivate

We discussed the prizes. She really wanted to go to a movie with three of her friends and get that candy, so we agreed that she needed 20 points for that prize.

- Going to a movie with three friends and getting candy **20**
- Going to the arcade with a friend **10**
- Getting frozen yogurt with Dad **5**
- Getting a manicure with Mom and a friend **50**

It was gratifying to see this going in a positive direction.

Step 7: Reinforce Progress and Increase Challenges

We met three weeks later to review results. Kara was successful at letting her mom leave her activities for a few minutes and now rated that a 1. She also did very well on the field trip and earned her 10 bonus points. She went to the movies with her friends and is now working toward the manicure.

So what's next? We discussed Mom leaving activities, driving away in her car to get a cup of coffee and then returning. Kara rated that a 7. She would get 2 points every time she did that, because it felt hard, and 10 bonus points for five times in a row of her mother leaving her at her activities.

We also discussed bedtime. This felt like the hardest for Kara but was the one thing her parents wanted most to change. Taking the cot out of her parent's bedroom and having her mom or dad stay in Kara's room until she fell asleep in her bed seemed like a good first step. The first night she did that would earn an automatic 10 points and a special prize in the morning. The next night 9 points, then 8, then 7, and so on. The first night is always the hardest, and then it gets easier. She would get 5 bonus points for five days in a row.

I emphasized the importance of consistency and suggested she listen to music in her room. We also reviewed how she needed to talk back to her worries.

Finally, Kara seemed ready to make a giant leap, and her parents were ready to support this.

"Things are getting better," her mom said, "but we still have more work to do."

Next Steps

Kara continued to work on her goals. Her parents learned to break the goals down and then gradually increase them. They understood the concept of challenging Kara but not overwhelming her. They worked on the sleep issue and were surprised at how quickly she was able to sleep independently.

This is common with sleep anxiety. The idea of sleeping alone is more anxiety provoking than the reality. When the child and the parents all agree to the goals, and parents are able to follow through, the step-by-step approach should work.

I often recommend doing this, the way Kara did, over a long weekend to start. Planning and agreeing when to start this is important. Parents have to be willing to set the limits, which can include doing things that affect their sleep, like bringing the child back to her bed.

Starting this on a long weekend when sleep was not an issue, having a good incentive, and using music quickly worked for Kara. As a result, her parents understood that under no circumstances should she go back into her parents' bed. This should not be thought of as a "treat" or something to do when Dad was traveling. Even if Kara is sick, Mom and Dad need to get their sleep and not take her into their bed.

Keep in mind: if kids go back to their parents' bed, this anxiety can easily return.

Dallan and Brendan's Story

Dallan and Brendan came into my office and started to tell me about Mary, their oldest of four kids. "She's 12," Dallan began, "and she's always been a very happy girl, but change has always been hard for her. She reminds me of what I was like as a child. We're here because it's hard to know how much of what she's going through is just normal 12-year-old stuff, and how much we should be concerned about. I was also sensitive as a child, and I never got help. I want Mary to learn some strategies to help her.

"Last year, going to school was often hard for her, and many times she'd go to the nurse with complaints of stomachaches, and I'd pick her up. In the back of my mind, I'd think she wasn't really sick. I'd get the call from the nurse usually when Mary was anxious about something. I tried to explain to her that her belly aches are really the worries, and she's not sick. She would cry in the nurse's office, begging me to take her home. She could literally scream about the pain in her belly. It broke my heart, so of course I would take her home."

Brendan interrupted, "She's a drama queen, Dallan. Let's face it. You get sucked right in."

Dallan responded, "You know that nurse. She always insisted I take her home. When I would say, 'Keep her in school,' they acted like I was being neglectful or something and demanded I take her home. And the nurse would always insist. Sure enough, when we got home, she always said her belly still hurt, but she sure didn't act like it. She could always eat anything and was usually hungry for lunch. She seemed very happy playing on the iPad or watching TV. When I'd ask her about her belly, she would say, 'It still hurts really bad.' If I tried to confront her about this and say, 'I don't think your belly hurts so much,' she would immediately scream about how bad the pain was. I know she likes drama, but what am I supposed to do? What if it really does hurt?"

Dallan described what they had already tried. "We took her to doctors, and she had all the tests. Everything's normal. They said it's just anxiety. She needs to be put on medication for her anxiety. So we started her on Prozac, but so far, it's not working, and she's starting to look like she's more distracted and a bit hyper. Medicine worries me; there has to be another way to help her. I secretly wished they'd find something wrong that we could treat, and all this would go away."

Mary's parents needed help understanding how treatment and medication can work together to help reduce anxiety. Yet knowing what kind of treatment is helpful and when to add the right kind of medication can feel overwhelming and confusing to parents.

"We took her to another therapist, and they did play therapy," Dallan continued. "I'm not sure what they did, but she loved going because they played games. Sometimes the therapist only had times to see her during the school day, so I took her out of school. She loved that. Every week we went there, but I have no idea what went on. I talked to her therapist, who was nice. She said they were working on her anxiety. But after all these appointments for over a year, and all this money, she's still crying at school, and I didn't see any change. She's been taking the Prozac now for a couple of months. My husband and I just felt we had to look at something else."

I asked Dallan to reflect on her own experiences.

"I remember feeling like she feels at school when I was her age. It was like a wave would sweep over me. It was very physical. I would feel hot and shaky and just feel like I had to go home. She says the same thing. I remember it like it happened yesterday. Change was hard for me too, but I never got help. I just had to deal with it."

I then asked Dallan to provide more details about Mary's experience at school.

"This year Mary started middle school, and I thought she'd be fine. She took a tour of the school last spring, and all summer, she seemed excited to go. The first week or two was fine, but then it all started again, only worse. She cries every night, saying, 'I can't do it. I can't go to school. Please don't make me go!'

"Then she cries in the morning and says she can't eat breakfast, her stomach hurts. Now she's breaking down and crying in school. I'm sure her getting to sleep late because she's so upset, and not eating breakfast, is only making everything worse. Everyone at school has been wonderful. When she gets anxious and starts to cry, she can go to the school counselor and stay there until she's ready to go back.

"This past week she had a couple of days where she didn't cry at school. I keep telling her she can cry at home, not at school, but then I don't want her thinking she can get attention for crying at home. It seems like she gets home from school and immediately talks about how hard it was and starts crying. I don't know what to do."

Dallan seems exasperated. "Did I say the wrong thing to her? It's so hard to know. I wonder, did I create this? But her sister, Julie, who's a year younger, is just the opposite. She's so independent. She has no anxiety. She'll go anywhere and do anything, not a care in the world. I think to myself, is this girl mine? It's great to see. I'm so proud of her. But, wow, she's so different from me. I guess she's more like her dad. My husband has zero anxiety. He is clueless when it comes to all this."

Brendan, who had let his wife do most of the talking, jumped in. "Mary is like you, and Julie is like me. I never had anxiety. I was always excited to go places. I went to camp all summer when I was a kid, every year. I love my parents, but I had a blast being away from them. I never missed them. I think both our kids should go to camp too, but this is where we disagree. I think we should just force Mary to get over this nonsense."

"Camp?" Dallan said. "Maybe Julie for a couple of weeks, but Mary hates camp. She went to day camp for a week and cried every morning, and after two days she stopped going. All that money we paid for it, down the drain. She likes staying home in the summer. Her cousins live close, and she plays with them. We go on vacation as a family, and she's fine, no stomach problems. She has a great time in the summer. She's just not a camp girl. She can't even do sleepovers with friends."

Brendan looked annoyed. "How are we going to help Mary if she can't do sleepovers? All her friends do it, and she always has to come home early. Remember last year when her class went away for two nights, and she cried every night, wanting to come home? She made it through, but other kids weren't crying like that. Maybe sending her to camp would cure her of this. She'd cry in the beginning but then settle down. I remember when I was a kid, there were always a few kids who were homesick in the beginning, but then they'd be fine and have a great time in camp. We have to get her over this."

Dallan raised her voice. "I can't do that to her! That would be torturing her. We can't just force her to go to sleepaway camp." She took a deep breath and continued. "I know we have to do something. I know when I went away to college, it was so hard for me. I ended up home the first year. I couldn't do it. I don't want that to happen to Mary. I know that's far off, but we have to help her and give her strategies. In so many ways, she's this happy, active kid, but this is a problem. Sometimes, I think I should just homeschool her. Then she wouldn't have to deal with all this stress. Don't you think kids are so overscheduled and pressured now? Homeschooling might give her relief from all this."

Brendan rolled his eyes and said, "I can't believe you're saying this. You two would kill each other if you had to homeschool her. Look at how much you fight now. Homeschooling would be the worst thing for both of you."

Then Brendan appealed to me. "We really have a great marriage. Honestly, it seems like Mary is the only thing we argue about. We're all fed up with this. Even her sister is angry and upset with Mary over this."

Brendan looked at Dallan, then back to me. "We need to tell you about the questions. She needs to know where we are every minute of the day. Every morning she grills us about when we're going to be home. If we're not going to be home, she needs to know where we'll be and for how long. I always tell her I'll be at work and that's the end of it, but with my wife, it can go on and on. Mary panics if we don't tell her."

Dallan chimed in. "Because I work from home, she's worse with me. It's like she wants me home all day when she's in school, and if I have to go into the office or even to the store, she gets upset and wants to know when I'll be back. It's like she worries about us if we're not home or something. Then the same panic happens when I have to pick her up somewhere. She needs to know what time I'll get there. Then she watches the clock, and if I'm a few minutes late, she panics. Now I've been trained to be perfectly on time with her or there'll be a crisis. I find myself getting anxious if I hit traffic or something."

Then Dallan's phone beeped. Brendan looked at me and said, "I guarantee you that's Mary. This happens constantly. When they're not together, the texting is constant."

Dallan quickly texted back. "Yup, that's Mary. She texted 'I love u, where r u?' She knows where we are. She has to check. If I don't return her texts, she panics. I always have to keep my phone on. I know she also expects me to text her when we're on our way home. He's right—it's constant. I guess I'm used to it. I don't think about it anymore, but it's actually stressful for me. I always have to be available to her, because I don't want her to get stressed. I know what that feels like, and I don't want her to have those feelings.

"I don't know if this is part of the change thing, but it's like she's younger than her friends. She's popular, and she does a lot of activities, but more and more, it seems like she doesn't want to grow up. It's like she hates the idea of puberty. When she got breast buds, she actually cried. Every time I try to talk to her about wearing a bra, she wants nothing to do with it. I think she wants to stay a child. She still sleeps with her doll. Her sister, Julie, on the other hand, is a year younger, but not only does she want a bra, she's bugging me about wearing makeup and shaving her legs. These two couldn't be more different."

Brendan nodded, but then said, "I know we've been talking a lot about Mary's anxiety, but wait till you meet her. She's popular, athletic, smart in school, and she's kind. She's the first kid to notice when another kid is sad or hurt. She's very sensitive. She's got the whole package, and ironically, in some ways, she has no anxiety. She had the lead last year in the play. She was Annie. She can sing and perform in front of a huge crowd of people, and she loves it. She's even running for student council. It makes no sense."

Brendan shook his head. "I can't figure it out. Here she is, crying at school and, at the same time, preparing her speech for student council and talking about tryouts for the next play."

Dallan agreed. "That's what's so confusing. She's so normal, and we know in a month or so, the crying will be totally gone, and she'll be fine. It's just that she shouldn't have to struggle like this every time there's a change. She needs strategies. I don't want her to go through life like this. We've provided her with a very stable life. Our family's great. We're really very fortunate, but her life can't always be like this."

I told the parents that Mary's life didn't have to be like this. They nodded hopefully, and we made plans for me to meet with Mary.

Mary's Story

As Mary settled in with her parents, she was a little hesitant but then began to express herself, echoing much of her parents' concern: "I don't know why I sometimes get so upset about school. It just feels so different being in middle school. I liked my other school, and I felt so comfortable there. This feels so big and loud, and I just get these strong feelings like 'I have to get out of here. I have to go home!' I get really hot and feel sick. My stomach hurts, and I get this shaky feeling, and I can't help crying. Sometimes when it's really bad, I feel like I can't get enough air. I can't breathe. My heart beats really fast. It's scary.

"I'm afraid all these bad feelings are going to come again. Sometimes I just feel like I have to get home. I can't stay in school another minute. I have to see my mom. Once I'm home, these feelings totally go away. When I'm with my family, I feel so happy. That's why I love summer so much. We're all together. I get to stay home. Everything's great. No worries."

She catches her breath. "Then school has to start, and we're not together. That's so hard to get used to. I don't worry something bad will happen to me. I worry something bad will happen to my mom and dad . . . I worry they'll be in a car accident, or something terrible will happen and they'll die. I know that sounds weird, but I worry I won't see them again."

I ask her to tell me more.

"When my mom's picking me up at my activities, I get so stressed out. I keep worrying until I see her, then I relax. And if she's late, I panic. I think the worst, and I can't help it. My mom doesn't understand this, but I like it better when we carpool and my friend's mother picks me up. I have no worries then. When it's my mom, it can be really hard. I also need to know where my parents are going to be every day. If my dad travels, until I know he's landed in the plane, I worry the plane is going to crash, so he has to text me when he gets on the plane and when he gets off. I wish my mom would just stay home all day. If she leaves home, I need to know when she's leaving, and she needs to text me when she gets home. I need to know she's okay. If she doesn't text me right back, I start to worry. I think something must be wrong. So I keep texting her until she texts back. She needs to keep her phone on when we're not together."

Mary continued. "I love the way things have always been. I have such great memories. I never want to lose my memories. My mother wanted to change my room because I'm getting older. I told her I liked my room just the way it was. She thought it was babyish. So she 'surprised me.' I came home one day, after being at my friend's house, and my bedroom was totally different. She got me all new furniture. I was so mad at her. I cried. I wanted my old furniture back. I begged her to get it back. She said it was gone. I couldn't believe it. I'll never see that furniture again. I got so angry, and then she got angry at me. She said I wasn't grateful. She thought I should be happy. But I never wanted new furniture. It makes me sad just thinking about it. I wish I could get my old room back. I hate surprises. I'm still so mad she did that."

Dallan was silent as Mary continued. "The other thing my mom does that drives me crazy, she wants to talk about my body changing. I don't want to hear about it. I want her to stop and leave me alone. I get mad at her every time she brings it up. She doesn't understand. I hate all these changes. I wish my body could just stay the same. I don't want to talk about it."

I asked her about her sister.

"Julie acts like she's a big teenager or something. She's so annoying. She acts stupid with makeup and all that. I don't want to hear about it. When she wants to put makeup on me, I get really mad at her. We used to have fun playing together. Now, especially when she's with her friends, she acts so different. They talk about boys and crushes. I hate it.

"My dad doesn't understand. He thinks I should be doing sleepovers like Julie does. I can't. I need to sleep with my parents. I know most kids don't, but I do. I would get too scared being in someone else's house. I need to be close to my mom and dad at night. That's just the way I am." She sighed as this session came to an end.

Mary was like a lot of kids with separation anxiety. She seemed happy and, in many respects, normal and well adjusted. When she was in her comfort zone of being with family and not coping with changes, she was free of anxiety. When triggered by some separation from parents or unexpected changes, however, panic could overtake her, seemingly out of nowhere.

Though her dad may not have accepted this yet, Mary was in crisis. What we all acknowledged was that this was very disturbing for the whole family. Even when things settled down and the anxiety abated, it returned with the next change.

In between periods of high anxiety, parents often learn to accommodate the lower level of separation anxiety by not challenging their child to do things they know will trigger panic. They accept things like texting with Mom, not wanting to sleep away from home, not wanting parents to leave home, asking questions about safety issues, and some clingy behavior, more the way a younger child acts. Parents assume this is "just the way she is" or that "she'll outgrow this."

In this case, Mary's mother had experienced many of the same feelings as a child and didn't want her daughter to go through what she had gone through.

So we were all ready to tackle strategies that I expected would help.

Step 1: Target Anxious Thoughts and Behaviors

Mary started by reiterating her worry that something bad would happen to her mom or dad. When asked about what bad things she thinks of, she paused, then said, "I worry they're going to get into a car accident or something like that. I worry they're going to die, and I'll never see them again." Her eyes welled up, and she started to cry. "Sometimes when I'm really worried, and I have to leave them, it feels like this is the last time I could see them, and I get so upset. I don't want to leave them."

Her parents looked surprised at the intensity of her feelings. They hadn't realized she was quite so worried about them dying. But of course it made sense, in a way. Why else would she become so hysterical at separation?

Mary continued. "I think I have to know where they are, just to make sure they're okay. I wish they would just stay home all the time, but if they go places, I need to know when they'll be home. If they're late, even by a few minutes, I start to worry, and that's when I get so scared and upset."

Then she looked at her parents and said, "That's why I need to know when you're coming, and you can never be late or it freaks me out."

Her parents seemed to begin to appreciate the depth of Mary's feelings as she continued to talk about how she hated change and aging, and the scariest inevitability of death.

She stated what we all realized: "I don't want to grow up. I want things to stay just the way they are."

Then she restated her fears about often not wanting to stay in school. "When I go to the nurse, I really do feel sick. I know my dad doesn't believe me. I hate when he makes jokes about me faking it. My belly really does hurt. At school I have to text my mom to make sure she's okay, and if she doesn't answer, I call her, and if she doesn't pick up the phone, I keep calling her until she does. I hate these feelings."

I explained that we could isolate those feelings and confront them.

Step 2: Rate the Anxious Behavior

Mary needed to identify her anxious thoughts and change them so she could "talk back" to her anxiety. Her thoughts about her parents' safety fueled her anxiety, so she really had to work hard at challenging her anxious thoughts.

How hard was it for her to talk back and challenge her anxious thoughts? How hard would it be to ignore these anxious thoughts when they came?

She rated her worries accordingly:

- Worrying that something bad will happen to my parents when I'm at school   7
- Worrying something bad has happened to my mom when she's late picking me up   10
- Worrying something bad has happened to Dad when he's traveling   6
- Feeling sad and upset about changing things in the house   5

- Worrying something bad has happened to my parents when they go out together   4
- Worrying something bad has happened to my parents when they go out together and are not home on time   10
- Worrying about changes   5
- Worrying something bad has happened to my mom when I know she's gone into the city   6

Then she rated how hard it would be not to do her anxious behaviors:

- Not knowing where Mom and Dad are each day 8
- Not texting Mom when I'm at school 7
- Not texting Mom when she is not at home 8
- Not texting Mom if she's late at pick-up 10
- Not texting Mom when I don't know where she is 8
- Not texting Mom when we're both home but in different parts of the house 3
- Not getting upset about changes in the house 3
- Talking about body changes 5
- Staying home when mom runs errands 5
- Not going to the nurse when I feel worried 8
- Not going home when I feel really scared at school 6

Step 3: Agree on Challenges to Work On

Mary looked at her list, and together we talked about what she could work on.

Everyone wanted to focus on her anxiety at school, since that was causing so many problems right now.

She agreed to work on five goals:

- Not going to the nurse at school
- Not calling or texting Mom from school
- Not texting Mom when she's not home
- Not asking Mom and Dad every day where they'll be
- Challenging her thoughts at school about her parents' safety

Next, we agreed it was time to begin the implementation stage.

Step 4: Identify and Teach Strategies to Practice

We discussed talking back to the worries and realizing that her worries about her parents were silly worries. She didn't like the term "silly worries"; she thought it meant she was being silly. So we talked about what she wanted to call her worries, and she decided to group them under the name "Brain Trickster," because they tricked her brain into believing false things and worrying.

We reviewed the reality: her parents were not sick, and they didn't do dangerous things, so the chances of something being wrong with them were very slim. So she needed to learn to talk back to the Brain Trickster: "My parents are fine. I will see them later. I am not going to be bothered by these worries. I am going to focus on being here and everything that's happening around me in school now. I am not listening to what the Brain Trickster is telling me. I will not be tricked. I need to ignore these worries, watch them fly by in my head. I can focus on being with my friends, learning from my teacher, doing my work at school, having fun at home. I can switch the worry channel off in my head because I'm the boss of my brain. I am smarter than the Brain Trickster, which lies to me when it says something bad happened to my Mom and Dad. I can listen to music and focus on happy things and not the worries. I can do this!"

She agreed to make a calm-down playlist of music she can listen to and sing with to help calm herself. After all, she is a little actress and loves to sing, so this was perfect for her.

She also made a calm-down list of things she can do that help her relax. At home:

• Draw
• Write stories
• Read
• Listen to music
• Sing and dance
• Do yoga stretches
• Play in the backyard
• Play games
• Watch TV

At school:

• Use her squeeze toy
• Focus on the teacher and her friends

- Remember they are brain trick worries
- If she needs to, take a break and get a drink of water
- Doodle on her doodle pad
- Talk back to the worries and let the thoughts fly out of her head

Step 5: Note and Chart Progress Made

Mary and her parents worked on making a chart and recording progress.

Her dad worked in computers, so he used a spreadsheet that included the date, her goals, her ratings, and her points. They agreed to keep it in the computer, and every evening they created a new spreadsheet with a flowchart showing progress. At this time, they would review her goals and her progress and add up the points she'd earned.

Step 6: Offer Incentives to Motivate

Mary's point system included more points for firsts as well as bonus points for repeated success:

- She would get a point every day she didn't go to the nurse at school, with a bonus 5 points when she didn't go five days in a row.
- She would get 2 points every day she didn't call or text Mom from school.
- If she called or texted and Mom said, "Talk back to the worries," Mary would get 1 point if she remembered to be in the here and now, use her calming list, and not call or text anymore.
- She would get a bonus 10 points for five days in a row of no texting or calling Mom from school.
- She would get 2 points when she didn't call or text Mom when Mom was not home.
- She would get a point every day she didn't ask Mom and Dad where they would be all day, with 10 bonus points for five days in a row.

Using points for days in a row of changing behavior is a powerful way to make the change stick. Mary was excited when we talked about her prizes. Based on her point system, her parents decided how many points she needed to get her prizes. Together they made the list.

- Go roller skating with friends **50 points**
- Go to the movies with friends **50 points**
- Have a sleepover **60 points**

- Make brownies **20 points**
- Go out to breakfast with Dad **25 points**
- Choose what Mom will make for dinner **10 points**

She was excited to begin working to get her prizes.

Step 7: Reinforce Progress and Increase Challenges

Mary came back two weeks later with her parents, and they had printed out their chart from her dad's spreadsheet. She was making progress.

She had earned points for not texting or calling Mom from school but had not yet gotten five days in a row. That had gone down from a rating of 7 to 5. She had gone four days in a row, so she was close. We discussed what had happened on the day that triggered her to text. Mary thought about it and then remembered: "In health class, we talked about diseases, and I started to worry that my mom might get a disease. I just had to text her to make sure she was okay." We then discussed how she could handle that if it happened again. I asked her what she could say to herself. How could she talk back to that worry? "I know my mom's healthy. She's not sick. I know it sounds silly now that I was so worried. I could have let the worry pass, ignore it, and focus on school and my friends. I also could have taken a break and gotten a drink of water. I just went right away to my phone to text her."

She had done a great job of not asking every day where her parents would be. That was down to a 2. She was proud to say she'd only been to the nurse once since we'd met, and she had been there for only a short time and returned to her classroom. Her parents praised her for this, and she earned a lot of points. Not going to the nurse was down to a 2, almost gone as an issue.

Not texting Mom when she wasn't home and Mary was home was still hard. She had some days when she didn't text and others when she texted once but didn't keep calling or texting. She rated that a 6. She still had to work on that one.

We looked back at her list, and she decided to work on some other goals since she was doing better. We added "Not texting Mom when we're both home but in different parts of the house," which was a 3. She also added to her list "staying home when Mom runs errands," which was a 5. She would get a point for each day she worked on those and 5 bonus points for five days in a row.

Mary was also excited to tell me she had already earned some prizes. She had gone out to breakfast with Dad, and she had chosen her favorite dinner, macaroni and cheese. She was also very close to having one of her bigger prizes.

All of us were happy that we were moving in the right direction. Her parents talked to the doctor who prescribed her Prozac, and they decided that since she was making progress, they would wean her off the Prozac. Her mother said, "We really don't think it's doing anything for her, and she now knows strategies and is able to work on managing her anxiety. We want to see if she can be okay without it."

It was agreed that they would continue doing the CBT every day without the medication. Mary was very happy not to be taking the medicine, which she said "tasted awful." For her, that was another reward for working on her goals.

Next Steps

Mary continued to make progress. When we discussed her "fighting" the anxiety, this was hard for her. Her parents were eager for her to "get angry at the worries."

She explained that she had a hard time doing that because she's not an angry kid. She really had no personal experience getting angry at anyone or anything in an extreme way. So getting angry at the worries was hard for her. What she found works was imagining a cartoon character running around getting all excited in her head, and she could say back to that character, "Calm down. I know you want to protect me, but everything is fine, so don't get so excited. Everything is fine!"

Talking back to her worries that way really worked for her. This is a good example of how the approach needs to be individualized. It's certainly not one size fits all. This example also shows how kids teach us what works best for them. We have to learn to ask them and listen.

Mary had one week when her anxiety was high, and she felt exhausted. Her parents considered putting her back on Prozac, but the following week was better, and Mary has continued to get better. After several months of CBT, Mom called with very good news: Mary was doing very well, and they saw no need for an appointment at that time.

Mary's story is a good example of how anxiety can go up and down. Learning how to manage anxiety takes time and practice. It also demonstrates that many children don't need to be medicated if they engage in CBT. The need for medication depends on the severity of the symptoms and the ability of the child to respond to treatment. It is not a black-and-white situation. Although Mary may continue to do well, she may also need a "tune-up" in several months or even years from now.

DSM-5 Guidelines

Separation Anxiety Disorder

The *DSM-5* identifies the diagnostic criteria necessary for a diagnosis. The assumption is that many readers will have children who meet some but not all the criteria.

A. Developmentally inappropriate and excessive fear or anxiety concerning separation from those to whom the individual is attached, as evidenced by at least three of the following:

   1. Recurrent excessive distress when anticipating or experiencing separation from home or from major attachment figures.

   2. Persistent and excessive worry about losing major attachment figures or about possible harm to them, such as illness, injury, disasters, or death.

   3. Persistent or excessive worry about experiencing an untoward event (e.g., getting lost, being kidnapped, having an accident, becoming ill) that causes separation from a major attachment figure.

   4. Persistent reluctance or refusal to go out, away from home, to school, to work, or elsewhere because of fear of separation.

5. Persistent and excessive fear of or reluctance about being alone without major attachment figures at home or in other settings.

6. Persistent reluctance or refusal to sleep away from home or to go to sleep without a major attachment figure.

7. Repeated nightmares involving the theme of separation.

8. Repeated complaints of physical symptoms (e.g., headaches, stomachaches, nausea, vomiting) when separation from major attachment figures occurs or is anticipated.

B. The fear, anxiety, or avoidance is persistent, lasting at least 4 weeks in children and adolescents and typically 6 months or more in adults.

C. The disturbance causes clinically significant distress or impairment in social, academic, occupational, or other important areas of functioning.

D. The disturbance is not better explained by another mental disorder, such as refusing to leave home because of excessive resistance to change in autism spectrum disorder; delusions or hallucinations concerning separation in psychotic disorders; refusal to go outside without a trusted companion in agoraphobia; worries about ill health or other harm befalling significant others in generalized anxiety disorder; or concerns about having an illness in illness anxiety disorder.

American Psychiatric Association. "Separation Anxiety Disorder." In *Diagnostic and Statistical Manual of Mental Disorders*. 5th ed. Washington, DC: American Psychiatric Association, 2013.

Chapter 6

Tap, Check, Count, Wash, Repeat

Obsessive Compulsive Disorder (OCD)

Obsessive compulsive disorder (OCD) is an anxiety disorder that causes people of all ages, including children and teens, to have distressing thoughts, or worries, that they cannot control. These worries cause them to feel an urgent need to perform certain rituals or rigid routines. The worries are obsessions, and the things they feel they need to do are compulsions. Children often feel they have to do these compulsions or something bad will happen.

Fortunately, OCD is very treatable, and there is much research supporting CBT as the most effective form of treatment. Specifically, the preferred approach is called exposure response prevention (ERP), which means the child practices being exposed to the OCD trigger and does not do the compulsion. With ERP practice, the feeling of needing to do the compulsion gradually disappears. This is how to become free from OCD.

One of my patients didn't know about OCD; she called her compulsions her "have to do's." Children with OCD usually think the "bad things" that could happen involve harm coming to themselves or their family members. These compulsions provide immediate relief from anxiety temporarily, but then soon they have to do them again and again. This cycle of obsessions and compulsions may take up hours of a child's time each day. OCD causes great distress and is confusing for children because they know they shouldn't be doing these compulsions, but they can't stop—the behavior feels out of their control.

Common obsessions are the fear of dirt or contamination, the fear of hurting others, the fear of thinking evil or sinful thoughts, intrusive violent or sexual thoughts, the need for symmetry or exactness, excessive doubt, and the need for reassurance. Common compulsions are repeated washing or showering, using excessive soap, repeated checking, avoiding touching things that are "dirty" like doorknobs or sticky substances, counting, arranging things, repeating tasks or words, making others repeat things, rereading, rewriting (writing over letters), rituals involving the keyboard or the Internet (having to go back and redo when typing, for example, or having to do certain things when the computer is turned on or off), touching, tapping, mental rituals to cancel out "bad thoughts," hoarding useless things, and seeking reassurance. The Children's Yale-Brown Obsessive Compulsive Scale is a useful reference to see a complete list of the OCD symptoms kids may have. It's also used as a reliable measurement of how severe the OCD is.

Up to 4 percent of children and adolescents have OCD, and most are diagnosed in childhood. That represents over one million children and teens. The disorder is often genetic, with one or both parents or other relatives having it. Usually by the time children are diagnosed, they report having had OCD symptoms for years. Many of these children and teens are high-functioning kids, good students, and athletes, popular, kind, and sweet. They are high functioning in every way, except they have OCD. Sometimes these kids resist treatment because having a "disorder" and needing help is a huge contrast with their self-image as normal, successful kids.

Some children have a sudden acute onset of OCD, sometimes accompanied by severe anxiety and motor or vocal tics. This type of OCD is thought to be caused by strep or another bacterial infection, known as PANDAS (pediatric autoimmune neuropsychological disorder associated with strep). This is controversial since the research is conflicting, and certainly more research is needed. There is no doubt, however, that a subset of kids with OCD very suddenly develop severe symptoms.

OCD can be extremely painful for children, making them feel trapped in a cycle of obsessions and compulsions that are overwhelming and confusing. For parents, family life can be much disrupted because OCD, like other anxiety disorders in children, can greatly affect the whole family, often turning day-to-day family living upside down.

With this as a backdrop, I present two illustrative case studies based on my patient experience.

Willy and Anna's Story

Anna called my office sounding desperate. She left a voicemail that ended with her in tears. She wanted my soonest available appointment because she felt so worried about her young daughter, Atalaya. I met with her and her husband, Willy, as soon as possible. They arrived early to the appointment, and once they came in, they began talking rapidly.

Anna started. "We are here because of our 7-year-old daughter, Atalaya. Something is really wrong, and we don't know what it is. She seemed fine up until ten days ago. Then she suddenly began worrying about germs and washing her hands all the time, saying things were dirty over and over again. We tried to talk to her about it, but it was like she couldn't hear us. We thought it would just go away, but instead it has gotten worse. We called you because it got to the point where she is now having a hard time using our bathroom. She woke up in the middle of the night and had to pee but she was hysterical about the toilet being dirty, the sink, the doorknob. She was crying that everything in the bathroom was too dirty. The poor thing ended up using the toilet squatting so she wouldn't touch the seat. She has never been like this before. She was the kid I used to have to remind to wash her hands."

Willy, looking concerned, added, "It is not just the germ thing. I get her and her sister up and dressed in the morning and take them to school. Getting her dressed has become impossible. She keeps saying nothing feels right, and she breaks down crying. I hate to say it, but she has worn the same loose t-shirt and loose flannel pants to school for the last week. She says these are the only clothes she can wear. She looks like she is wearing pajamas to school. I'm sure the kids and teachers are going to start to notice. In addition she is worried about her fingerprints. She feels like she has to wipe off her fingerprints. I know this sounds weird, but she is frantic about it."

Anna added, "I wash her clothes every night. I try to get her to wear different clothes, but she just panics and cries. She also told me that now she can't use the bathroom at school. She is holding it in all day. And she thinks even our bathroom is contaminated. She's washing her hands so much they are red and chapped. She asks a lot of questions over and over again, and my husband realized now she's trying to get us to repeat things. At first I thought she wasn't hearing us, but she keeps asking us to say the same things again and again. What has happened to our little girl?"

"She also asks the weirdest questions," Willy added. "It feels like it's all day long now. She says things like, 'I touched the chair and then I touched my mouth—is that okay? Should I wash my hands?' I say, 'No, don't wash your hands,' but she runs into the bathroom and washes them anyway. Lately, and I know this sounds disgusting, but she has started spitting, thinking she is getting rid of dirt in her mouth. If I don't answer her questions, or if I tell her to stop spitting, that there is nothing in her mouth, she gets really angry and melts down. Putting her to bed has become a nightmare, between the questions and the washing and what I need to say to her eighteen times before she lets me leave her. It's taking almost an hour just to get her into bed. She has these things we have to say to her over and over, and she has to wipe her fingerprints, and she is doing things over and over again. She is getting to sleep so late, and we are all exhausted."

Willy looked down at his hands. "I admit I get angry at her. I just want her to stop this. She has a younger sister, and it feels like she's being neglected because all our time is being spent with Atalaya. We are so worried and don't know how to help her. She was never like this. She was a happy, normal child. A month ago I was thinking she could grow up to be the president. Now I worry she may never be . . ." Willy suddenly stopped, and his eyes watered up as he said "normal."

Anna took Willy's hand and said, "We just don't know how to help her. I don't know what's going on, but she is getting slower and slower. Willy is right. It's such a struggle. I dread bedtime. My stomach gets tight once dinner is over, knowing what we face. By the time she gets to bed, it's so late, I know she must be exhausted. I'm exhausted and angry. I know I shouldn't, but I feel so angry. She says such mean things to me when she's like this."

"And she wakes up in the middle of the night and ends up in our bed," Willy said. "Then I end up in her bed. It's crazy! She was always such a good sleeper. We used to just tuck her in at night, and she would go off to sleep. In the last two weeks, everything has changed; we don't know what to do. We feel either sorry for her or angry at her or both. We don't know whether to punish her or just comfort her. It's so confusing. None of us are sleeping, and her sister is wondering what's going on."

Anna then said, "We started reading about OCD on the Internet, and we think that's what she has, but what do we do about it? I worry about what's happening at school. I can't imagine that she's not worried there, too. I don't want to tell her teacher. We don't know what to do. We just want to help her, but instead of it getting better, it seems to be getting worse."

I could see on their faces how hopeless and defeated as parents they felt, not being able to help their child. We agreed that the next step would be to meet with Atalaya.

Atalaya's Story

Atalaya began to relate her concerns: "I have so many worries all of a sudden. I don't know what's happening to me. I think everything is dirty, and I have to wash my hands a lot. I keep thinking about germs, like they're everywhere, and now everything is germy. Bathrooms really scare me now because everything feels so dirty in the bathroom. It feels like pee is everywhere. Sometimes I have to change my pants because I think there is pee on them. Sometimes I want to wash my leg after I use the bathroom because I think maybe pee is on my leg, but I know it isn't. At first it was just the school bathrooms that were dirty, but now even my bathroom at home feels germy. I wish I never had to use the bathroom ever again. I try to hold it as long as I can, but then I have to go. I hate taking showers now; it feels like I have to do more and more to get clean. Sometimes I feel like as soon as I am clean, something happens to make me dirty again. It makes me so mad. I just want to scream. Nobody understands how bad this feels!

"Then I have the worry about fingerprints. I feel like I have to rub them off. Someone could be seeing my fingerprints and will then try to hurt me. Everything I touch, I have to rub."

It was easy to feel Atalaya's pain as she continued. "I also have a really hard time getting dressed. None of my clothes feel right. I try to put them on and have to take them off because they feel so, . . . so uncomfortable.

I can't stand it. I don't know why, but I have only a few clothes that feel 'right.' The rest I can't wear. Mommy and Daddy don't understand. I can't help it. Sometimes I just cry and cry because it feels so bad. I can't wear the clothes I used to wear. I just can't. Everything takes so long now. I am always late, but I have so many things I have to do in the morning now, and my parents keep yelling at me to hurry up. I can't go any faster. I have to make sure everything is right, and I have to wash."

I asked Atalaya about bedtime. "At night my worries get worse," she said. "I hate bedtime. I have all these things I have to do before I go to bed. Turn the light switches on and off, fix my stuffed animals a certain way, close and open my drawers, check the closet and close the door, and then brushing my teeth is a big deal, and the washing. Then when finally I get into bed, I feel like my parents have to keep saying, 'Good night. I love you. Everything is okay. See you in the morning. I love you. I love you.' Four times, or if that doesn't feel right, six, eight, ten times. Last night they had to say it sixteen times. It can't be an odd number, because I know that is bad luck, and something bad will happen. They get mad at me sometimes, and then they have to start over. If they won't do it, I can't get to sleep. I can't. Something bad will happen if they don't do it. They have to say this before they leave me at night. I don't know why this is happening to me."

Clearly feeling exhausted, Atalaya wrapped up her story: "At school sometimes I can forget about it all . . . until I have to go to the bathroom, or I touch something that's dirty, and then I get worried all over again. There are two boys in my class who are really dirty. One of them picks his nose, and the other picks at his ear. I can't even walk by them without feeling like I have to wash my hands. Sometimes even just looking at them from my desk makes me have to wash. I am so glad there's hand sanitizer in the classroom. I keep using it over and over again. Some kids asked me why I was wearing my pajamas to school. I couldn't explain to them. I didn't know what to say. I don't know why. I told them it wasn't pajamas and walked away. Sometimes I worry I must be going crazy. I want this all to stop."

I explained that if we worked together, we could begin to make it stop. I explained the seven steps, starting with Step 1.

Step 1: Target Anxious Thoughts and Behaviors

What are Atalaya's anxious thoughts (obsessions)? Atalaya and her parents made a list of all her worries.

- Germs and pee and poop getting on me
- Feeling really dirty, so dirty it just sticks on me and won't go away
- Not being able to get clean enough
- Getting poisoned by putting the wrong thing in my mouth
- Wearing clothes that feel so uncomfortable and that yucky feeling won't go away
- Fearing something bad will happen to me or my family
- Fearing someone will get my fingerprints and hurt me

What are Atalaya's anxious behaviors (compulsions)?

- I have to wash my hands a lot, with at least four squirts of soap over and over, or use hand sanitizer.
- I have to spend a lot of time in the shower. I have to wash every part of my body over and over again an even number of times and tap the soap.
- I can't turn the shower on or off; I need my parents to do it because the shower handle is too dirty to touch.
- I can't use the school bathrooms. They are way too dirty.
- It is getting really hard to use the bathrooms at home. There is only one that I can use now, and I can't sit on the toilet. The seat is too dirty. After I use the toilet, I have to wash my hands and sometimes my legs because I worry I got pee on me.
- Sometimes if I think something touches my mouth, I need to ask about it to make sure it is okay. And then I usually have to wash my hands and sometimes even spit to get the dirt out of my mouth.
- When I touch some things at school, I have to use the hand sanitizer. I always have to use the hand sanitizer if I go near two of the boys in my class who are really dirty.
- I sometimes have to ask my parents if they washed their hands, especially when they are cooking.

- I can't wear most of my clothes. They don't feel right.
- My parents have to say good night to me in a certain way and a certain number of times or else I can't go to sleep.
- I have a lot of things when I brush my teeth. I have to put just the right amount of toothpaste on the brush, then tap it against the sink four times. Then I have to brush each side top and bottom an even number of times. When I'm done, I have to spit an even number of times and then tap the toothbrush against the sink and then I'm done.
- I have to wipe all my fingerprints away, especially at night, because that's when bad things happen.

Atalaya's parents listened patiently as she made her list. Before it was over, her mom had tears in her eyes. I asked Atalaya to leave the room as I could see her mother was starting to cry. Her mom broke down. "It's so hard. I'm exhausted. I get mad at her. None of us has gotten enough sleep. We haven't told anyone about this. Her sister keeps asking what's wrong. We don't know what to tell her. When she's up at night doing all these things and I get mad at her, she starts crying and screaming and wakes her sister up. Our whole family feels like it's been turned upside down."

We discussed how OCD is really a family illness, because everyone becomes affected. We also discussed telling the other kids that their sister is not feeling well and is having a lot of worries that she can't control. They needed to know that she was getting help and this would get better. I reassured Atalaya's mom that getting angry is a normal reaction, and that we would soon be working together to fight the OCD, which would make things feel more positive at home instead of a struggle with each other.

Atalaya came back and joined us as we talked more about how we would work together to get rid of her OCD. Atalaya looked relieved that she had shared all her worries and felt, perhaps for the first time, that her parents understood, and that she really wasn't going crazy—she just had this thing called OCD. I let her know that lots of great kids have OCD and that she would learn how to "kick it out" of her head. Since she is a good soccer player, this made her laugh.

She was ready to do the work and go on to the next step.

Step 2: Rate the Anxious Behavior

Next Atalaya read through the list and rated each compulsion or behavior on a scale of 0 (easy) to 10 (impossible) based on how hard it felt to not do what OCD was telling her to do.

- Not washing my hands when I feel they are dirty 9
- Using two squirts of soap when I wash instead of four 7
- Washing only once in the shower, not over and over again 5
- Turning the shower on and off myself 7
- Using the school bathroom 10
- Going into the school bathroom 8
- Using my parents' bathroom without sitting on the toilet 3
- Sitting on the toilet 7
- Using the bathroom downstairs 8
- Not washing my legs when I think I got pee on them, even though I know there is no pee there 4
- Not seeking reassurance about getting something dirty in my mouth 6
- Not spitting when I feel like I have dirt in my mouth 4
- Not using hand sanitizer when I think I touched something dirty at school 4
- Not using hand sanitizer when I come near the dirty boys 5
- Not asking my parents to wash their hands 3
- Wearing clothes that feel uncomfortable 8
- Not doing the bedtime rituals with the lights and stuffed animals 8
- Not having my parents say good night to me that certain way 9
- Not doing the tooth-brushing things 8

Since sleeping had been such a problem, as it often is in children with anxiety, we decided to add it to our list.

- Going to bed by myself, without needing Mom or Dad to stay with me 8
- Staying in my bed throughout the night and not going into Mom and Dad's room 10

With the identifying and the rating accomplished, we were ready to work on certain challenges.

Step 3: Agree on Challenges to Work On

I explained that we needed to pick some things that she could work on to fight OCD. Atalaya was beginning to learn that OCD needs to be seen as something outside her that she can fight and get rid of. The more she fights OCD, the weaker it gets, and the stronger she gets. I explained to her that OCD is a liar, telling her to worry about dirt that isn't there and telling her she has to do things she doesn't have to do. She can say "no" to OCD, and that is what will make her better. I also reinforced that lots of kids have OCD; she was not alone, she was not going crazy, and she would get better. I told her she was going to kick OCD really hard right out of her head.

Thinking about what to work on was something we all did together. Atalaya became fidgety and suddenly seemed to look like a much younger child as she leaned into her father. She was scared, afraid it would be too hard to do this. We focused on the things on her list that were not rated too high. I reassured her that I wasn't going to force her to work on something she didn't feel ready to work on. She could choose with us what she'd work on, and I would help her with making her OCD go away.

Her hands were not only cracked but also had been bleeding from so much washing. I knew that hand washing had to be brought to the top of the list. Her little hands really hurt. I was also concerned that they could become infected. I let her know that whatever she decided to work on, she would be earning points toward prizes for doing this work. She was excited about the idea of prizes. I listed everything that was not too hard, and Atalaya led us in choosing what she'd work on.

Not washing when she felt her hands were dirty was rated very high, but we needed to help her with her cracked skin. She agreed to try to work on it, but how? We needed to break it down into steps that were not rated so high. With hand washing, sometimes kids' hands look red not because they are frequently washing their hands but because when they do wash, they use too much soap, or they don't dry them because they don't want their clean hands to touch the towel. Atalaya was both washing too frequently and using a lot of soap, which explained why her hands looked so bad. Plus it was winter, and the cold air made them even drier.

She agreed to use two squirts of soap instead of four. She rated that a 7, very hard. Because her hands looked so sore, however, we encouraged her to work on this.

She agreed to work on exposures concerning the hand washing. We made a list of "dirty" things that she agreed to touch without washing her hands afterward, and she rated them:

- Doorknobs in her house (but not the bathroom doorknobs, which was too hard). She thought that would be a 6.
- Not washing after she touched the TV remote, the computer mouse, and her iPad. That was a 7.

She understood that to do an "exposure," she needed to practice touching these things over and over again and not washing, until she felt like she didn't want to wash. Her anxiety level would go up at first, but then it would go down. This is the work of fighting OCD. I explained that it is called exposure response prevention and that it's the greatest tool in overcoming OCD.

She also agreed to a few additional goals:

- Not wash after each meal and snack. She rated that a 5.
- Not use hand sanitizer when she looked at or walked by the boys in her class that OCD was telling her were dirty. She rated that a 5.
- Work on wearing different clothing. This was a priority because of the obvious social effects. Again we had to break it down. She agreed to wear one shirt that she had not been wearing because she thought it was uncomfortable and didn't feel right. She rated that a 6.

Next, although she was most anxious about bedtime compulsions, we needed to talk about them since they were so disruptive to the family. Also, kids with OCD and anxiety need their sleep. If they don't get enough sleep, their symptoms can be much worse. We agreed to start with her limiting the bedtime verbal ritual with her parents. Her parents were extremely frustrated with having to say these bedtime phrases over and over again. She agreed that they could say them twice instead of four, eight, or twelve times. She rated Mom and Dad saying the bedtime ritual twice as a 6. We also discussed her listening to an audiobook of her favorite story. She loves *Diary of a Wimpy Kid*, so listening to that made her feel good. She agreed that her parents could leave her with the book on a timer, to turn off automatically, and that she could turn the book on again if she woke up in the middle of the night. We talked about "silly worries" and her need to focus on the book and remember that she is safe in her bed. We also added an additional bonus reward she could get in the morning if she stayed in her bed all night. Dad agreed to make M&M pancakes. That was a great treat for Atalaya.

We agreed we were making progress and proceeded to the next step.

Step 4: Identify and Teach Strategies to Practice

The first strategy is to label the OCD and recognize that OCD is something she can fight and not give in to. Learning to recognize that her worries were OCD would help her see them as things she needed to "boss back." She liked the idea of thinking about it as a game she could win and OCD could lose. When OCD was telling her she had to do her compulsions, she had to learn to say "No" and remember that she is the boss of her brain. She needed to change the way she was thinking about these obsessions and compulsions. Her parents were also learning how to help her with this. Their role became like coaches, encouraging her to fight OCD and supporting her efforts through praise and incentives.

The second strategy is to resist doing the compulsion. She had to practice not doing what OCD told her she had to do and realize that nothing bad happens. This was hard work for her and felt very uncomfortable at first, but she learned that it got easier and easier the more she practiced. We talked more about how to do exposures, where she intentionally triggered OCD and then resisted doing the compulsions, again and again, until she no longer felt like doing them. Some of her behaviors, like getting dressed, were difficult to do exposures with since they happened only once a day. She was starting to understand that any time she could do exposures, they would help her fight the OCD.

Willy and Anna had to learn strategies that could help them parent

Atalaya through this difficult time. They needed to be reminded that this was a process and would take time. They had also researched more about PANDAS and had taken Atalaya to her pediatrician. While waiting for the strep test results, they were learning how to stay focused on the agreed-on goals and how to coach Atalaya to fight the OCD and reinforce this work with positive incentives. Having a plan of action made them feel optimistic, less helpless, and ready for the next step.

Step 5: Note and Chart Progress Made

Charting is extremely useful for several reasons. First, it gave structure to Atalaya's CBT plan. The chart would list specifically everything we had agreed that Atalaya would work on, so the goals would be clear. Second, the chart would remind Atalaya to work on her goals. She was a busy girl. With school, homework, sports, and other activities, it might be easy to forget about the need to *fight* her OCD and not just give in to it. Looking at the chart reminded everyone, including Atalaya's parents, of the work that needed to be done every day. Third, it gave Atalaya an opportunity to chart not only the work she was doing, but more importantly, her progress. By keeping track of how hard these things were, using our 0-to-10-point scale, she would see how that number goes down as she practices, until it is a 0 and she can cross it off the list. Having such a clear measurement of her progress as she did this work would help keep her motivated and positive about the process. And last but not least to Atalaya, her chart would help her keep a running total of the points she had earned toward her prizes.

Her chart needed to be simple and easy to work with for both Atalaya and her parents. Together we discussed how to do this. She would list what she was going to work on each day, check it off when it was done, and rate how hard it was. Atalaya would work with her parents to design the chart. They also discussed where they would keep it. Atalaya didn't want her friends to see it when they came over, so they decided to put it in her drawer next to her bed. They also decided on a time each day to review the chart together. After dinner made the most sense, so they agreed to do it then.

Now, on to the all-important incentives.

Step 6: Offer Incentives to Motivate

Every day that Atalaya worked on her list and recorded her anxiety rating, she earned a point. Since she was working on eight things, she could earn up to 8 points a day. If her parents noticed that she was fighting OCD on things that were not on her list, or if she told them she fought OCD, she could earn bonus points. For example, the first week of doing this, not only did she wear a different shirt, but she earned bonus points for wearing different pants.

But what did she want to cash her points in for? This was the fun part. Atalaya and her parents discussed what she would like to earn and came up with a fun list. They then figured out how many points she needed to get to earn these prizes. Given her young age, she needed to earn prizes quickly to keep motivated.

Her point and prize list:

- Gift card for bookstore **50 points**
- Breakfast out with Dad   **35 points**
- M&M pancakes for dinner **25 points**
- Baking with Mom   **15 points**

- Sleepover and movie with two friends   **50 points**
- Ice skating with a friend **20 points**
- Swimming at the Y with a friend **25 points**

Atalaya was now very excited to fight the OCD. She was ready to show results.

Step 7: Reinforce Progress and Increase Challenges

After a couple of weeks, Atalaya was proud to show off her chart. In the meantime, her test for strep came back positive, and Atalaya was diagnosed with PANDAS. She started taking antibiotics. She made progress with her goals and was proud to show me that her hands were looking much better. We reviewed her chart, and she had gone beyond her goals. She was now earning points for one squirt of soap when she washed, since after a few days, two squirts became easy (rated a 0), so she reduced the soap even more. Touching the remote, iPad, and mouse and not washing were now 0, so we crossed that off her list. Doorknobs were still difficult, so she needed to keep working on that. Touching them without washing was a 3, and we wanted it to be 0. She was able to walk by the "dirty boys" without sanitizing her hands, so we crossed that off her list. Not washing her hands after eating was still a 3, so she needed to keep working on it. Having Mom and Dad do the bedtime ritual twice was easy, so we discussed not having them do it at all. She said that would be a 6, but she was ready to work on it.

Since we had crossed off things that she was no longer worried about, we needed to add some more things. We agreed to start tackling some of the bathroom difficulties. She agreed to take faster showers (fifteen minutes or less) and to turn the shower on and off herself. She said that was now a 7. She also agreed to sit on the toilet in her parents' bathroom, rated a 6, and to use the other bathroom in the house, a 7. She now understood the power she had to fight OCD and was excited to talk about the prizes she had earned.

Anna and Willy were pleased. Anna said, "It is still hard. She is making progress, but we have more work to do. We are fighting with her less and so proud of her because we see how hard she's working. I never in my wildest dreams thought we would have to go through something like this, but having a plan and seeing the progress gives us hope."

We agreed to meet again in a few weeks to monitor her progress and increase the goals.

Next Steps

Atalaya was able to make very quick progress. She went from experiencing acute onset OCD to feeling completely better within weeks. Her mother said, "We have our daughter back!" Her parents are convinced it was the antibiotic that made a huge difference for her, and they are now firm believers that their daughter has PANDAS. They also realize that no matter what the cause, OCD responds very effectively to CBT. They know to be aware that if her symptoms come back, it may again be strep. We all hope that she will not have a relapse, but they know to call me if she does. Atalaya now refers to her OCD as "the time when my brain went crazy" and is so glad it's gone. She has also learned that if the symptoms return, she needs to immediately start working step by step to control them.

Don and Lori's Story

Don called me with concerns about his son's increased worries, and he seemed eager to meet as soon as possible.

"My son Barry is 14 and really struggling," he began. "He is doing weird things, and he came to me and his mother last week and announced that he has OCD. I was frankly shocked, because he is an athlete and loves nothing more than being covered in dirt. And if you looked at his bedroom . . . to put it nicely, he's a slob. I always thought OCD was about hand washing and keeping clean. That's not my son. He insists he looked OCD up on the Internet, and he's convinced he has it. His mom and I are divorced and share custody. She was as surprised as I was by this, although we both have been worried about him. We researched OCD, and I guess it can include a lot of different things. I don't know if he has OCD, but I know my son needs help."

I agreed to set up an appointment with Barry's parents. They agreed that they could easily meet together. Although some divorced parents prefer separate meetings because they have strong conflicts with each other, these parents thought it would be better to meet together.

Both arrived on time and explained that they had been divorced for almost ten years and shared custody. Lori, Barry's mother, started. "I have known something has been wrong for years. He has always been a worrier and had these weird things he had to do at night and things he made me say at bedtime. I talked to my pediatrician about this several times, and she always said that if it doesn't interfere with his functioning, leave it alone. Well, now it's interfering. My son's suffering with lots of weird things he feels he has to do over and over again. And his guilt . . . he's guilty about everything. Not only that, but he's now spending hours on homework. Nighttime is so difficult, with him spending so much time doing God knows what, but he's not getting to sleep until very late. Then getting him up and to school is such a struggle. He also asks questions over and over again: 'Is this okay, is that okay?' It feels like he is constantly seeking reassurance even about silly things. As much as I try, he's been late to school, and I've been late to work. This has to change!"

Don added, "I see the same thing. I try to talk to him, and it doesn't work. He's going to bed later and later, and mornings are a struggle in my house, too. When he said he has OCD, I don't know if that's what it is, but he's right, something's very wrong, and we need help. He's been so irritable, and when I see him up way past his bedtime in the bathroom, I try to get him to bed, and he screams at me and says, 'Now I have to start all over again.' I have no idea what he's talking about. Nothing I do seems to work. Last night he was crying and saying, 'I have to do this. Leave me alone. I have to do it.' It was after midnight. I have no idea how to help my son, but I know he needs help."

It was clear that I needed to meet with Barry as soon as possible.

Barry's Story

Barry seemed to welcome the opportunity to express his thoughts: "I finally told my mom and dad what's been going on in my head, but I didn't tell them everything. I've had this thing in my brain that tells me to do things for a long time, but lately it has gotten so much worse. I have to count just about everything now: the steps I take, brushing my teeth, chewing my food, opening and closing my locker, everything has to be in multiples of four.

"It's so annoying. I can't stop it. If I don't do it, it feels like something very bad will happen. It could be that I will fail a test or worse, something bad could happen to my parents. I thought I was going crazy until I looked it up on the Internet and found out that it's OCD. I read stories about other kids who count and have to read over things again and again, and they worry just like I worry. I thought I was the only one who had all this stuff going on in my head. What a relief to read other kids saying they do exactly what I do."

Barry described worrying about everything. "Sometimes I think I did something bad, like cheat on a test. I know I didn't cheat, but then I worry that maybe I did. It's crazy. I feel guilty about all the things I did wrong in the past. I can't get them out of my head. It's all worse at night. I keep asking my parents all these questions to help me stop worrying. I know they're getting frustrated with me, but I can't help it! They yell at me in the morning because I'm so slow. I don't mean to be slow, but I have to do all these things over and over again. Nothing is easy anymore. And at night it takes me a long time to get to bed and finish my homework. I have to read things over and over again. I used to like to read, and now I hate it. Then in bed, I sometimes get these bad thoughts. I get the thoughts during the day too. Thoughts that I am going to stab someone like my mom or dad or even my dog. I am afraid of knives, scissors, anything sharp. I feel like I might do something bad. I need help. I can't get this stuff out of my head. My parents don't understand. I hate this OCD!"

Barry agreed to meet with his parents and me so we could all work together to help him.

Step 1: Target Anxious Thoughts and Behaviors

Barry made a list first of his worries (obsessions) and shared it with his parents.

- Something bad will happen to me or my parents if I don't do things a certain way or in multiples of four.
- I will go crazy and become a mass murderer.
- I did something very bad.
- I will do something very bad, like stab someone or my dog.
- I'm a bad person.

Then he made a list of his anxious behaviors (compulsions), which he would later rate based on how hard it would be to resist doing them (0, easy, to 10, impossible).

- Counting and doing things in multiples of four, including:
  Brushing my teeth

Washing my face

Having to wash everything at least four times in the shower

Turning lights on and off

Opening and closing doors and drawers

Opening and closing my locker and backpack

Chewing

Stepping (I have to always start with my left foot, and I can't stop walking unless it has been an even number of steps.)

Rereading

- Seeking reassurance when I think I did something bad or when I doubt what I'm supposed to do:

From my dad

From my mom

From my teachers

From my friends

- Avoiding:

Sharp objects (knives, scissors)

Reading

As is often the case, while his parents listened to him make his list, they were surprised and saddened by the burden Barry was carrying. His father said, "Barry, I can't believe you're still able to do everything you're doing with all this in your head."

His mother agreed. "Now I understand why you were doing these weird things and why homework has been such a struggle. It all makes sense now."

With this heightened understanding, we moved on to Step 2.

Step 2: Rate the Anxious Behavior

Barry next assigned rating codes:

- Not counting and doing things in multiples of four   **8**
- Brushing teeth   **7**
- Washing face   **3**
- In the shower   **6**
- Turning lights on and off   **7**

- Opening and closing doors and drawers 5
- Chewing 8
- Walking 5
- Rereading 8

- Opening and closing locker and backpack 6
- Not seeking reassurance 8
- Not avoiding sharp objects 10
- Not avoiding reading 6

Next, it was time to address the challenges.

Step 3: Agree on Challenges to Work On

Barry and his parents had already started learning about OCD. Barry needed to change the way he was thinking about the disorder and realize that it was something he needed to fight and not give in to. Barry knew that there was no special power in doing these things, but he felt he couldn't stop because not doing them made him so anxious. We discussed how difficult everything was for him due to his OCD and focused on the most important obsessions and compulsions to work on. Getting to bed earlier and getting to school on time was very important to Barry's parents. Don said, "Barry, you're being so selfish. Don't you realize you're making your mother and me late for work because of all this? We are all so stressed in the morning. It's not fair!"

Barry looked sad, and tears swelled in his eyes. "Selfish? I'm sorry, Dad. Don't you realize it's because of you I have to do these things? I feel that if I don't do them, something terrible will happen to you or Mom. I can't stop it."

I explained that this is OCD, and that Barry is not intentionally caus-ing these problems; he feels out of control. Our goal was to get him back in control and rid him of the OCD.

Barry agreed to work on several behaviors:

- Not rereading. Even though he rated his rereading compulsion at an 8, it was important that he reduce this because of the effect it was having on his life. He used to be an avid reader, but now that had stopped. Homework was taking so long because of his rereading. He was frustrated by it and wanted it to stop.
- Not seeking reassurance from teachers. Barry was a good student and was

aware that his questions to teachers were starting to annoy them. He liked his teachers and wanted them to like him, so he was very motivated to stop this. He knew the questions he asked were silly, like asking over and over again what the homework was or when the next test was. He was also aware that even his friends in class were getting frustrated with him. He asked these questions because he kept doubting himself. Obsessive doubting is a common OCD symptom.

- Not seeking reassurance from his parents.

- Taking less time in the shower. This was important to him because his shower compulsions made his morning routine take too long. He had been late for school and was making his parents late for work.

- Not opening and closing his locker four times. He wanted to stop this because he was worried kids were starting to notice, and it was weird.

As Barry bought into our approach, he was more prepared for the next step.

Step 4: Identify and Teach Strategies to Practice

The first thing that Barry needed to learn was that OCD was lying to him, telling him he had to do these things when he didn't have to. He needed to strengthen his insight into the fact that these behaviors had no special power to prevent or cause bad things. Life doesn't work that way. He needed to take the power out of OCD by seeing it as something outside himself that he had to resist. He also needed to be reminded that many great kids have OCD. He wasn't losing his mind, and he could get rid of his OCD. He also needed to learn to "talk back" to OCD when he doubted himself and wanted to seek reassurance. He needed to remind himself that he knew the answer and didn't have to ask more questions. Then he needed to focus on the here and now and not on his obsessive thoughts. This is how mindfulness helps with OCD: focus on the experiences in the moment, not on the OCD thoughts—let them go.

His parents also had to understand the disorder so that they could help him. They had to learn that trying to be rational with him when he is stuck with OCD only escalated his anxiety. They also had to remember that as hard as all this was for them, it was harder for Barry. These behaviors can have a great impact on the whole family, and sometimes it's hard to remember that OCD behavior is not your child's choice; it's something they feel they "have to do." Barry didn't want to be doing these things; he felt he had no choice. Working together as a team, we would change that.

Rereading is a very common OCD symptom. Sometimes it's driven by just having to read something a certain number of times; sometimes the anxiety is that everything has to be understood perfectly, so the rereading occurs until it just feels "right." This is not to be confused with children who have ADHD or a reading learning disability, who really need to reread because they do not understand the content of the material. Barry felt he had to reread until he understood everything perfectly. But he needed to change the way he was thinking about this. He didn't have to know it all perfectly. All the details aren't important. There are a few strategies to help with rereading. One is listening to audiobooks and reading along with them. Barry needed to remember that the longer he went without rereading, the easier it would be. He had to read and listen to the book without rewinding the audio. When an audiobook was not available, he could try reading out loud to help him resist rereading. He could make a game of it, by trying to see how long he could go without rereading and then trying to go longer the next time. He was a very competitive kid, so this seemed like a great strategy. When he rereads, he needs to think that OCD wins, and he loses. This was a strategy that clicked with Barry. Because he's a boy who always likes to win, OCD didn't have a chance against him.

To help Barry work on not seeking reassurance from teachers, we needed more information. How many times was he asking teachers questions to seek reassurance? Reassurance questions are those he knows the answer to but that his obsessive doubting makes him feel he needs to ask again and again to make sure he's right. Barry said he easily asked four or five questions in each class, with less in math, usually one or two, and science more, up to about eight questions sometimes. He sheepishly admitted that yesterday he had asked the science teacher four times when the next test was. The fourth time he asked the same question, the teacher was clearly angry. He also noticed, for the first time, that some kids were rolling their eyes and laughing as they started to notice.

The strategies he used included remembering that the questions were OCD, and that he knows the answers. Then he needed to limit himself to a certain number of reassurance questions per class. He agreed to no questions in math, three questions in science, and two questions in all the other classes. Knowing he had a limit and keeping track of it would make him more aware of each question, and he would want to think a lot before he asked because he wouldn't want to use up his questions too fast. This would help him ask fewer questions, and eventually we would work on him asking no OCD questions in school.

For not seeking reassurance from his parents, it was agreed, since this was so frequent, that he would have two times during the day when he could seek reassurance. The first was at breakfast, and the second was after dinner. When he wanted to seek reassurance at other times, he needed to postpone his questions until the designated times. This was easier than saying he couldn't seek reassurance at all. That was too hard for Barry right now. When Barry's reassurance time came, he most likely would not need to seek reassurance, because his urge for it will have passed. This is a good step toward no reassurance seeking.

For the shower, he agreed to wash himself twice, not four times. Talking back to OCD meant reminding himself, "I am clean enough."

For the locker, he agreed to opening and closing twice instead of four times to start, telling OCD "No" when he got the urge to do it more.

Step 5: Note and Chart Progress Made

Barry agreed to keep a simple chart in his phone for his OCD work.

For the rereading, he would keep track of how long he went without rereading. To keep it simple when he's reading, he would just record the date and then how long he was able to read without going back and rereading (two paragraphs, one page, three-quarters of a page, etc.), and at the end of all his reading for that day, he would rate it based on how hard it was not to reread, from 0 (easy, no rereading) to 10 (couldn't resist at all), with 5 meaning he reread about half the time.

For the shower, he would record just the date and how many times he washed, keeping it simple for him.

For school, he decided to use a laptop that he had with him all the time. Using a notes program, he would record how many times he asked

OCD questions and how many times he opened and closed his locker. This would keep it easy for him to remember as well as private.

Barry also agreed to use a point system.

For the shower, he would get 5 points if he washed only once, 3 points if he washed twice, and 0 points if he washed more than twice.

For the OCD questions at school, he would get 2 points if he asked no OCD questions in math, 0 if he asked one or more questions; for science, since that was his hardest, he would get 5 points for no OCD questions, 4 points if he asked one, 3 points if he asked two, 2 points if he asked three, and 0 points for more than three. For all the other subjects, he would get 3 points if he asked no OCD questions, 2 points if he asked one, and 1 point if he asked two—any more than two, and he would get 0 points.

For seeking reassurance from his parents, he would get 5 points for seeking reassurance in the morning only at the designated time, which they identified as five minutes after he eats breakfast, and 5 points for saving his later questions for the five minutes after dinner they had agreed on. If he slipped and asked an OCD question, his parents would quickly say "OCD" and not answer the question. If he was able to refocus on something else not related to the OCD and resist continuing to seek reassurance, he would still get his points. We also agreed, however, that if he absolutely needed reassurance and couldn't resist, his parents would reassure him, but he would not earn any points.

For his rereading, he would get 5 points every day he worked on it and showed less rereading overall than the day before, 4 if it was the same, 1 point if he tried and was using the strategies, and 0 points if he didn't try.

Since his parents were divorced and he went back and forth, keeping the chart in his phone, which he always had with him, made this simple. Every evening, they totaled up his points for the day.

But what about incentives?

Step 6: Offer Incentives to Motivate

Barry was excited to get in on this discussion. We realized what hard work this was going to be for him, and his parents wanted to offer him rewards for his effort in fighting his OCD.

Barry quickly announced what his parents already knew, that he wanted new basketball sneakers. He also wanted to go to sporting events with his dad and maybe a friend. His father makes his favorite meal, homemade pepperoni pizza, so he put that on his list too. With Mom, he loves her carrot cake and enjoys going to breakfast with her.

It was decided:

- Sneakers **50 points**
- Tickets to college basketball games with a friend **30 points**
- Ticket to a professional sporting event with Dad **100 points**
- Pepperoni pizza made by Dad **20 points**

- Carrot cake made by Mom **20 points**
- Breakfast out with Mom **20 points**

And now on to the final step . . .

Step 7: Reinforce Progress and Increase Challenges

After three weeks, Barry and his parents were ready to meet again. He had been working hard and making progress. He had earned his sneakers, breakfast with Mom, and pizza from Dad.

His chart showed progress, with his numbers of difficulty down. These numbers were important because they told us how hard it was for Barry to resist these compulsions. His most recent daily chart showed the following numbers.

- Reassurance morning, 0. He no longer needed reassurance in the morning. Great accomplishment!
- Reassurance evening, 6. He still needed to seek reassurance in the evening. The urge was still there.
- Shower, 0. He no longer felt the need to keep washing, but he was still doing it twice.
- Rereading, 5. He was still struggling with this one; it had improved, but he needed to keep working on it.

- Teacher reassurance, 3. This was much better but still needed more work.
- Locker, 2. This was almost done, but occasionally he was still doing the opening and closing.

Next we had to increase the challenges.

- Reassurance seeking in the evening, which he wanted to keep working on, 6. It now seemed easy for him in the morning but still difficult in the evening.
- Shower, washing only one time, 3. It was easy to wash only twice; now the goal was to wash only once.
- Teacher reassurance, 3. Decreasing his reassurance seeking was much easier than when he had started, so it was time to increase the goal. The goal now was no reassurance in his classes except science, which was the hardest, so he is allowed two OCD questions in that class only.
- Rereading, 5. Not rereading continued to be difficult, so we decided to keep those goals the same.

Now he also wanted to add some other OCD goals, including not counting steps. Since it always had to be an even number of steps, he would do an exposure of intentionally walking an odd number of steps. We did that in the office: he got up and took five steps and then sat down. His anxiety level went up to a 7, but after ten minutes, he was at a 0, no anxiety. He agreed to practice this every day and rate it. To chart not counting steps throughout the day could be too tedious, so we agreed that he could just rate himself at the end of the day. If he didn't count at all, that would be a 0; if he counted all the time and didn't resist, 10; if he counted about half the time, 5. At the end of the day, he would earn 10 points for not counting steps at all, 9 points for not counting most of the time, 7 points for counting half the time, 3 points for trying and resisting many times, and 0 for not trying or for resisting very little. He was on the honor system, but it was clear that Barry couldn't lie about this since he feels too guilty. He was an excellent reporter. We now planned to meet again in a few weeks, but he was really making excellent progress and reducing his OCD symptoms.

Next Steps

Barry continued to work on his OCD. After a couple of months, he was clearly making progress, but it was slow. Even though we attempted to work on his intrusive violent thoughts, to take the power out of the thoughts, he still couldn't do any exposures to sharp objects. He avoided all knives and scissors and was greatly bothered by these thoughts. In addition, he felt his anxiety was really interfering with his ability to concentrate at school. So he had a consult with a child psychiatrist, who added medication to his treatment (I refer patients for medication when appropriate but don't prescribe myself). With medication, his progress doing this work was much more rapid. He was better able to apply the skills he had learned and was feeling less anxious. We continued to meet once a month to review his progress and to agree on new goals.

His father said, "He is much better, and we are so proud of him. The work he has done to manage this OCD has been so hard. He really is a strong kid!"

DSM-5 Guidelines

Obsessive-Compulsive Disorder

The *DSM-5* identifies the diagnostic criteria necessary for a diagnosis. The assumption is that many readers will have children who meet some but not all the criteria.

A. Presence of obsessions, compulsions or both:

Obsessions are defined by (1) and (2):

1. Recurrent and persistent thoughts, urges, or images that are experienced, at some time during the disturbance, as intrusive and unwanted, and that in most individuals cause marked anxiety or distress.

2. The individual attempts to ignore or suppress such thoughts, urges, or images, or to neutralize them with some other thought or action (i.e., by performing a compulsion).

Compulsions are defined by (1) and (2):

1. Repetitive behaviors (e.g., hand washing, ordering, checking) or mental acts (e.g., praying, counting, repeating words silently) that the individual feels driven to perform in response to an obsession or according to rules that must be applied rigidly.

2. The behaviors or mental acts are aimed at preventing or reducing anxiety or distress, or preventing some dreaded event or situation; however, these behaviors or mental acts are not connected in a realistic way with what they are designed to neutralize or prevent, or are clearly excessive.

   Note: Young children may not be able to articulate the aims of these behaviors or mental acts.

B. The obsessions or compulsions are time-consuming (e.g., take more than 1 hour per day) or cause clinically significant distress or impairment in social, occupational, or other important areas of functioning.

C. The obsessive-compulsive symptoms are not attributable to the physiological effects of a substance (e.g., a drug of abuse, a medication) or another medical condition.

D. The disturbance is not better explained by the symptoms of another mental disorder (e.g., excessive worries, as in generalized anxiety disorder; preoccupation with appearance, as in body dysmorphic disorder; difficulty discarding or parting with possessions, as in hoarding disorder; hair pulling, as in trichotillomania [hair-pulling disorder]; skin picking, as in excoriation [skin-picking disorder]; stereotypies, as in stereotypic movement disorder; ritualized eating behavior, as in eating disorders; preoccupation with substances or gambling, as in substance-related and addictive disorders; preoccupation with having an illness, as in illness anxiety disorder; sexual urges or fantasies, as in paraphilic disorders; impulses, as in disruptive, impulse-control, and conduct disorders; guilty ruminations, as in major depressive disorder; thought insertion or delusional preoccupations, as in schizophrenic spectrum and other psychotic disorders; or repetitive patterns of behavior, as in autism spectrum disorder).

Specify if:

With good or fair insight: The individual recognizes that obsessive-compulsive disorder beliefs are definitely or probably not true or that they may or may not be true.

With poor insight: The individual thinks obsessive-compulsive disorder beliefs are probably true.

With absent insight/delusional beliefs: The individual is completely convinced that obsessive-compulsive disorder beliefs are true.

Specify if:

Tic-related: The individual has a current or past history of a tic disorder.

American Psychiatric Association. "Obsessive-Compulsive Disorder." In *Diagnostic and Statistical Manual of Mental Disorders.* 5th ed. Washington, DC: American Psychiatric Association, 2013.

Chapter 7

Scared to Death
Specific Phobias

All children have fears, and many of these fears are normal. Young children are often afraid of the dark or supernatural creatures, like ghosts or witches, and older children often fear bad things happening to them, like natural disasters. When a child develops a phobia, it's typically severe and persistent and affects normal life. Rather than getting better or growing out of it, kids with phobias often feel more frightened and avoidant over time, not less.

Children having a phobic reaction are in a "fight or flight" sense of panic. Their bodies respond as if they're in great danger when they are not. Their muscles become tight, and adrenaline is released, often causing physical symptoms, including rapid heart rate, nausea, chest pain, dizziness, and shortness of breath. Children having a panic attack like this may also become disorganized in their thinking and have difficulty processing what's happening to them.

Talking to a child in this state of intense anxiety is usually not helpful and can actually make things worse. They can't take in what is being said to them, and they are highly sensitive to being criticized. This is not a teachable moment—they are too far over the top with anxiety to process rationally what is being said to them. The best thing to do to help them is to focus on relaxation strategies and to rationalize only after they have calmed down.

Although all cases of phobia are unique, the examples in this chapter are representative. They focus on phobias related to dogs, thunder and lightning, and bugs.

Suma and Larry's Story

Suma and Larry came to my office very concerned about their daughter. Suma explained, "We are here about our 8-year-old, Ellen. We have three kids, all girls, and she's our middle child. She always seemed so happy-go-lucky, and in many ways, she's a normal kid. I would have never thought we'd find ourselves getting help for her, but here we are. Ellen has developed a severe, intense fear of dogs. She is petrified of them. In our community, this is a major problem. Most of her friends have dogs. Most of our neighbors have dogs. Dogs are everywhere. So she's severely limited by this fear. Ellen can't go on most play dates because there are dogs. Riding her bike is now out of the question. She can't even walk to the bus stop. She is basically housebound because of her fear."

At first, Suma hadn't wanted to accept her daughter's condition and would force her to go out and do normal activities. "That was until two weeks ago," she continued, "when we were bike riding together. It was a beautiful day, and we were talking and laughing side by side until she saw a dog. It was a little tiny dog, on a leash, all the way across the street from where we were riding. Ellen freaked out. She started screaming and crying and actually fell off her bike, she was so scared. I realized this was now a safety issue. I could imagine, God forbid, her running into traffic if there was a dog around. She becomes totally out of control, reacting and not thinking at all. Later, she feels so bad about it she cries. She knows it's irrational. Now I feel like I can't take the chance of having her outside if a dog might come around. I don't trust her to stay safe."

Suma then mentioned another fear that was also getting out of control: "She's afraid of thunder and lightning. She was always sensitive to noise, but instead of this getting better, it's getting worse."

She then looked at her husband and said, "I worry Larry is making it worse by praising her for her great knowledge about weather. I think it's gotten way out of hand."

Larry looked defensive and quickly jumped in. "She loves the computer, and it's a great learning tool. Our little girl knows more about weather patterns than a meteorologist. I got her lots of books on the weather, and she devoured them. She checks the current weather conditions and the forecast on the computer several times a day. If you want to know anything about the weather in this area for the next seven days, she has it memorized. She even did her science project on the weather. How can all this knowledge be a bad thing? Who knows, she may grow up to be a famous meteorologist on TV."

Suma interrupted. "Larry, it hasn't helped. If anything, she's worse." Suma then turned to me and said, "My husband is a scientist. He likes to think Ellen's following in his footsteps. I know knowledge is good, but this is out of control. The more she learns and studies weather forecasts, the more frightened she becomes if a storm is coming. If there are clouds in the sky, she doesn't want to go outside. On cloudy days, I literally have to struggle with her to go to school. Now with all her 'knowledge,' it could be sunny out, but if she thinks a storm could be coming, she's afraid to go outside. Her teacher says that if it's cloudy out, she spends a lot of time looking out the window and is distracted. On sunny days, she's fine. It's just like with the dogs. When there's thunder and lightning, she goes into a complete panic. She runs into the basement, huddling in a corner, away from any windows, covering her ears, often crying until it's over. In the middle of the night, if there's a storm, she runs into our bed and stays there, scared to death. Soccer season is starting, and she loves soccer, but I know, as soon there's a cloud in the sky, she's not going to want to leave the house. And what are we going to do about summer camp? Keep her home every time there's a chance of rain?"

Suma caught her breath and stated the obvious: "We clearly need help with this."

Larry added, "Don't get us wrong. She is a sweet kid and a joy. Other than this, she's our easiest kid; I can't believe she's gotten so extreme with all this. She has lots of friends, and her teachers love her. She's very smart and does well in school. Maybe she's too smart? I thought more information would help her to be less afraid, but maybe my wife's right. It certainly has gotten worse. I don't know the answer. We just need to know how to help her."

This sense of frustration led these caring parents to ask their daughter to meet together with me.

Ellen's Story

Ellen seemed mature and poised as she started to express her feelings: "I know dogs are cute and all, but they really scare me. I don't know why. I get so scared when they are near me. I just freak out. I can't help it. I guess I think they're going to hurt me, bite me. I feel like dogs can just get so out of control. I can't explain it. I just really get so scared. Even if they're on a leash, they might get off the leash. I just don't feel safe. I don't think dogs like me. Three of my friends have dogs, and I can't go to their houses to play. Even if they put the dog in another room, I'm still scared it will get out."

She took a deep breath before continuing. "When I was riding my bike the other day, all of a sudden I saw a dog being walked across the street. I started crying and screaming and got so scared, I lost control of my bike. I jumped off the bike and scraped my arm and leg. I can't ride my bike now because there are too many dogs around. I wish there were a place where no dogs are allowed, but I don't know of any place like that. I wish there were no dogs in this whole world, and then I would be fine. I don't hate them really. I just can't stand being anywhere near them."

Ellen then elaborated on the other big fear: thunder and lightning. "I get really scared that maybe there could be a tornado or a hurricane and we'll all die. That's how it feels when the sky starts to get dark, like we could die. People do die from lightning and tornadoes and hurricanes. I've read about all the damage they can do. It could happen to us. It's possible. When I know there's a storm coming, I feel like it's going to happen, that this could be it. I just get so scared. Nature can be unpredictable, you know. If there's thunder and lightning, forget it. I can't be outside. I have to go down in the basement and cover my ears until it's all over. Of course you never want to be near a window if a storm is coming. I think about this every day. That's why I always check the weather. I need to be prepared. If there are clouds in the sky, I check the weather reports again, and if there's a storm coming, I need to know when and how bad it's going to be and for how long. I've learned all about the weather and how to track storms, sometimes before I even see the weather report.

"If I had three wishes," she concluded, "there'd be no dogs ever, no storms ever, and every day would be sunny. That would make me so happy."

After hearing Ellen's words, I explained my recommended strategy, to use the seven steps. We agreed to set up the next session together to start working on Ellen's fears.

Step 1: Target Anxious Thoughts and Behaviors

First, we specified the different phobias, starting with the fear of dogs.

Ellen's anxious thoughts were hard to identify because she quickly moved from 0, being relaxed and happy, to 10, being in a panic. It seemed she instantly became filled with paralyzing fear. Rationally, she knew that dogs may not want to hurt her, but when she was faced with a dog, her thinking changed. She needed to first become more aware of her anxious thoughts about dogs, so she could challenge them before she automatically jumped to panic, oblivious to rational thoughts.

Ellen's anxious behaviors included:

- Total avoidance of friends' homes if they had a dog
- Not walking or riding her bike outside
- Avoidance of any setting where there could possibly be a dog, which in her community meant almost everywhere
- Crying, screaming, and running away in a panic if she saw a dog

Next, we addressed the phobia of thunder and lightning.

Again, she was uncontrollably afraid that something terrible could happen when a storm approached. Her fears included a hurricane or tornado that would kill people, or lightning that would strike her or her family. Although she was convinced that every storm could be fatal, she needed to understand that these were irrational thoughts that shouldn't trigger panic. We needed to work on greater clarity regarding these thoughts so that she could "talk back" to them and replace them.

Her anxious behaviors included:

- Checking the Internet to monitor the weather every morning, afternoon, and evening

- Avoiding being outside when clouds were in the sky and she feared a storm might be coming
- Not wanting to go to school on a cloudy day
- Seeking reassurance from others that a storm was not coming
- Reading everything she could about weather, storms, and other weather-related topics such as natural weather disasters
- Frequently looking out the window at school, making sure no clouds were in the sky
- Not being able to sit near a window at school, for fear lightning could strike her
- Not being able to go outside when it rains, for fear she's in danger

When a thunderstorm actually struck, her anxious behaviors included:

- Hiding in the basement away from windows
- Holding her ears
- Sometimes crying in fear
- Needing to sleep in her parents' bed
- Being unable to go outside

Next, it was time to address our rating system.

Step 2: Rate the Anxious Behavior

We went through all the behaviors on her list and asked her to rate how hard it would be, from 0 (easy) to 10 (impossible), not to do these things. She listened and then folded her arms, looking straight at her parents. "I'm sorry," she said. "I can't do any of this. It's too hard. They are all a 10. I can't change the way I feel. I'm too scared. Isn't there some medicine I can take to make this go away?"

At this point, it was very important to calmly assess the situation. I reassured Ellen that although there was no magic pill for this, we could make these scary feelings go away by working together. We broke down her challenges one at a time. First we looked at the dog phobia. I asked her parents if they knew of anyone who had a nice, sweet, mellow dog that we could work with. It should not be an active, playful puppy. It had to be a dog that they could see often, ideally daily, to work with. Ellen and Larry thought about it and then came up with a friend's dog, Sophia. She was 10 years old, very calm, and loved kids. Perfect. Ellen also knew Sophia, and she didn't used to be scared of her, but since this dog phobia had taken hold, she was even afraid of Sophia.

Ellen needed to challenge her irrational thoughts about dogs, but first she had to recognize them. This was hard for her, but she needed to know that these false beliefs fueled her anxiety.

She began to list these fearful thoughts:

- I am going to be attacked by Sophia.
- The leash could break, and Sophia will run after me.
- Sophia is going to hurt me.
- Sophia is going to bite me.
- Sophia is going to jump on me and knock me down.

We then discussed whether it was likely that Sophia would do these hurtful things. Ellen didn't even have to think about it. She knew Sophia was a sweet, gentle dog and would never hurt her. Her mom joked that Sophia was not a hungry wolf on the tundra; she was a spoiled golden retriever that lived like a queen. Ellen laughed and was on the verge of understanding that these worries were "silly worries," not based on what's real.

She then repeated the rational thoughts that she needed to tell herself, what she had to say in her head to talk back to her silly worries:

- Sophia is a nice, gentle dog and doesn't bite.
- The leash is strong and won't break; even if it does break, Sophia won't hurt me.
- Sophia likes kids and likes me and is happy to see me. That's why her tail wags so much.
- Sophia is a cute, soft dog who always looks like she's smiling.

We discussed where we could start in desensitizing Ellen to dogs, but we needed Ellen to guide us. I asked her a few questions, and then asked her to rate the difficulty, how high her anxiety would be.

- Can we walk by Sophia's house and look at her behind their front door? Ellen rated that a **1**.
- Can we have Sophia's owner, Mrs. Lee, walk across the street with Sophia on a leash? Ellen rated that a **4**.
- How about you walk by Sophia when she is on a leash and sitting? Ellen rated that a **6**.
- How about petting Sophia when she is on a leash, sitting, and your mom or dad is right with you and you just quickly touch Sophia? Ellen looked serious and said immediately an **8**.
- Touching Sophia when her owner has her sitting, on a leash, and covers her mouth? **6**.
- Riding your bike across the street from Sophia when she is on a leash? **7**.
- Putting food in a bowl for Sophia and watching her eat when you are away from her? **7**.

Now Ellen had told us where we should focus with her dog phobia. A rating of about 4 in her anxiety level would be a good place to start.

Next we addressed her storm phobia. Again, Ellen said everything was a 10, and she felt totally overwhelmed by this fear. We worked on the cognitive aspects. She knew her fears were irrational. I asked her to tell me her anxious thoughts and together we would work on replacement thoughts.

She listed her anxious thoughts:

- I see clouds, and a storm is definitely coming.
- I need to know if a storm is coming so I can be prepared and protect myself.
- If a storm comes, I could get struck by lightning and die.
- If a storm is coming, it could mean a deadly hurricane or tornado, and we can all die or lose everything.
- These storms could destroy our house.
- The louder the noise from the lightning, the more dangerous it is for me. If it's too loud, it will hurt my ears, and it means something bad is going to happen.
- Being outside or near a window when it's raining is very dangerous, and something bad could happen to me.

Then she listed her replacement thoughts, or as we called it, "The Truth about Storms":

- Clouds are not a message that a storm is coming. Many times there are clouds and no storm.
- I don't need to check the Internet. If a storm is coming, I will be okay.
- I'm safe if a storm is coming, and I don't need to hide in the basement.
- The chance of getting struck by lightning is very, very small.
- The chances of a tornado or hurricane coming where I live are very small.
- If a major storm is coming, my parents and teachers would be notified and know what to do. It is not something I need to prepare for.
- The loud noise of thunder is not connected to any danger.
- The chances of being struck by lightning by being near a window or walking outside during a storm are extremely small.

Once she has challenged these thoughts, she has a better mindset for rating the behaviors:

- Not checking the Internet at all   10
- Checking the Internet only in the evening   5
- Not seeking reassurance when there are clouds in the sky   6
- Not going into the basement when there is a thunderstorm   7
- Not covering my ears when there is a thunderstorm   5
- Not going into Mom and Dad's bed during a storm at night   10

- Walking outside during a storm   9
- Walking near a window during a storm   7
- Not crying or screaming during a storm   4
- Not complaining about going to school when it is cloudy or a storm is predicted   5

Now we were ready to tackle the phobias head on.

Step 3: Agree on Challenges to Work On

Ellen reviewed all she had written about her phobias, and we looked at actions that were not rated too high.

For the dog phobia, she first agreed to work on walking outside and looking at Sophia from across the street, where Sophia would be on a leash. Ellen would need to practice with Sophia as much as possible to reduce her anxiety. After each practice session, she would rate her anxiety level on a scale of 0 (no anxiety) to 10 (I can't stand it). For each session, her anxiety would go up, but then it would go down. When her anxiety was down, she could stop the session. She was reminded that the more she practiced, the faster her fear would go down until she was no longer afraid. When this was no longer hard, we would increase the goal to getting closer to Sophia with Sophia still on the leash, until Ellen could eventually pet the dog.

For the storm phobia, Ellen agreed to try several goals:

- Check the Internet only once a day, at night.
- Not complain about going to school on a cloudy day.
- Not seek reassurance when it is cloudy.
- Not cry when there is a thunderstorm but challenge her thoughts.
- Not cover her ears when there is a storm.

In addition, she agreed to work on gradually exposing herself to the sights and sounds of storms. She would download the sounds of thunder and wind on her iPod and listen to them. She also agreed to watch YouTube videos of thunder and lightning. At the local science museum, there was an exhibit about thunder that created a loud noise, and Ellen agreed to go to that with her father and not cover her ears.

We were seeing results as we began to implement strategies.

Step 4: Initiate and Teach Strategies to Practice

Ellen was taught how to challenge her anxious thoughts, talking back in her head with her replacement thoughts. For instance:

- Use mindfulness to experience what was happening around her and not rush to catastrophic expectations about what would happen if there were a thunderstorm.
- Practice staying in the here and now, where she is safe and in no danger.

- Focus on the feelings of rain falling on her and the sounds of rain and even of thunder. Closing her eyes, she could imagine these sensations and feeling calm. In addition to challenging her thoughts, she could work on desensitizing herself to the sights and sounds of storms. She had to stop running away from the feelings they provoked.
- Use calming activities to help her relax, including music, drawing, and reading.

We were getting there.

Step 5: Note and Chart Progress Made

Ellen and her mother drew up a chart that listed her goals and her ratings of how hard it was to practice these exercises.

Step 6: Offer Incentives to Motivate

As is usually the case, Ellen was very excited about earning prizes for doing this work. We agreed on a point system where she would earn one point every time she practiced working on her goals and two points when she moved up her goal to the next step.

We then discussed what she wanted to earn. She was eager to earn craft supplies (she loves making bracelets), special time with Dad going out for breakfast, special time with Mom baking cookies, and having breakfast for dinner. (She loves pancakes and waffles, and having them for dinner is a special treat.)

Mom and Dad looked at her wish list and decided how many points she needed:

- Craft supplies **30 points**
- Breakfast with Dad **25 points**
- Baking cookies **20 points**
- Breakfast for dinner **15 points**
- Sleepover and pizza with two friends **50 points**

Ellen was eager to earn her points.

Step 7: Reinforce Progress and Increase Challenges

Ellen and her parents came to meet four weeks later, and we reviewed her chart. It was filled with decorations and lots of stickers. Each sticker equaled one point, and she had clearly earned a lot of points.

She had been working very hard with Sophia on the dog phobia. For instance, every day after school, she had a "play date" with Sophia. She had graduated, step by step, from walking across the street from Sophia on a leash all the way to petting Sophia and giving her a treat when she was sitting. They were fast becoming good buddies as Sophia had learned to expect Ellen's play date as well.

When Ellen was even more comfortable with Sophia, the next step would be to go out and be exposed to other dogs. Ellen rated this a 6, much better than when we had started. She said, "I think I'm not so scared of dogs anymore. Sophia is fun to play with."

With the storms, she had done well with checking the Internet only once a day. Our goal was to get her to stop checking it at all. I suggested she move to checking once a week. Ellen's smile disappeared, and she looked worried. "No, I can't do that," she said. So I suggested checking twice a week on Sunday and on Thursday. She agreed to that and said it would rate a 7 on her anxiety scale.

She'd been watching videos of storms, and that was now "easy." She had also been listening to the sounds of thunder on her iPod, and she had gone to the science museum to listen to storm sounds. She said that both were also easy.

She did well with not complaining about going to school when it was cloudy, but one day when it was raining, she had not wanted to go to school. So we needed to help her with that when it was raining.

Unfortunately, unlike with the dog phobia, exposure to her weather-related fears was dependent on when there were thunderstorms, which were not that frequent. There had been only two thunderstorms since we'd last met. The first storm had been harder for her than the second. During the first one, she hadn't covered her ears or gone to the basement, but she had cried and hadn't been able to go near windows. During the second thunderstorm, she hadn't cried and had been able to walk by a window. She was making progress, but there was more to work on.

Ellen was also proud to show me her list of prizes and seemed very motivated to keep progressing. Hopefully, there would be more nonthreatening thunderstorms and friendly dogs for her to practice with.

Next Steps

Ellen's parents were able to work together and help Ellen face her fears, and she continued to make progress. After the most recent rain shower, she emailed me with great pride: "I was outside in the rain and not afraid. Yea!"

We continued to meet once a month. She's learned not to run away from her fears but to practice facing them.

Lenny and Tara's Story

Tara and Lenny came to meet with me because of their concerns about their 13-year-old son, Sam. "Sam is a great kid," Tara began. "He has Asperger's, and I always say he's our gift from God, just the way he is. He's sweet, gentle, and kind. There's not a mean bone in this kid's body. He has his quirks, for sure, but we love that he's different. However, the one thing that is really getting in his way lately is his fear of bugs."

Lenny added, "Flying bugs, to be specific. Show him a huge furry spider, and he couldn't care less, but a little flying moth, and he's in a panic. Makes no sense. He has had different fears in the past, fear of the dark, fear of monsters in his room, fear of being left alone, but they all came and went. This fear of bugs isn't going anywhere. I think it's even getting worse."

Tara agreed. "He's so scared of flying insects that now he's avoiding lots of things. Every day, it's something new. He won't go outside to play with his friends in the neighborhood. He won't go out for recess at school. He won't play in gym class if it is outside—you name it, he won't do it. He has become a huge homebody, which is not like him."

Lenny continued. "At first I thought he was staying in just to play those stupid computer games, but no. I took the games away, thinking that would get him to go outside, and it made no difference. He still wouldn't budge. He refuses to go out of the house. He is so afraid of bugs, he runs like a maniac from the house to the car when we are going somewhere, and he does the same thing when we get somewhere. He's out of the car but running into shelter like he's being ambushed. I have even seen him flapping his arms to keep the bugs away. I tried to say, 'Buddy, you got to stop that; it looks really weird.' You know what he said? 'Dad, I have Asperger's. I don't care how it looks.'"

Tara was shaking her head. "This kid is smart as a whip, and he has an answer for everything. He's right. He doesn't care what anyone thinks, and I guess there's good and bad to that. Sometimes I wish I had Asperger's, so I wouldn't worry so much about what other people think."

"Tara, this isn't about Asperger's, or other people," Larry said. "I don't want Sam scared so much of the time. He used to love nature, hiking and playing outside. He was the kid who could play outside with a stick and walk around picking flowers in the backyard by himself for hours. Now, in seconds of being outside, he's in a panic. Sam needs to be outdoors. He needs the fresh air and exercise. Since this whole thing got so much worse several months ago, I'm sure he's put on weight. He stays home sitting and eating snacks, instead of being out, running around with the other kids. It's not healthy for him. I feel like I've tried talking to him till I'm blue in the face about bugs, insects, nature, you name it. He listens and seems to learn, but then he goes right back into fear mode when it comes to going outside. You would think our house was surrounded by killer bees."

It was time for Sam to see me.

Sam's Story

He began, "I have entomophobia, or insectophobia. Take your pick. It means fear of bugs. I have a very bad case of this disease. I hate bugs. You don't have to tell me about bugs. I know all about them. I have thirty-four books on bugs. I know their names, what they look like, how they mate, what they eat." He told me there are some nine thousand different kinds of insects in this country and 6 to 10 million species on the planet. He also reported that the evolution of winged insects is very controversial. Some researchers believe that their wings evolved from gills; others disagree. He believes in the gill theory himself, although he said that there's not conclusive evidence to support it 100 percent.

"Last year I did a science project on bugs," he told me. "I am the bug expert in my school and still I suffer from entomophobia. I don't think anyone is going to be able to help me. Therapy just won't work with me. I think it's okay if I'm afraid of bugs. There are worse things to be afraid of, actually. Do you know how many different phobias there are? I've studied that too. I love my mom and dad and my sister, Alice. That's really what's most important, right? There are lots of things I'm not afraid of too. So why don't we just leave my little fear of bugs alone, okay? So let's just forget about this therapy stuff, okay? I talked about it for months with another therapist, and it didn't help. I can accept that I have this phobia, but I wish my parents would leave me alone and not keep bringing me to therapy."

I encouraged Sam to continue. "I love the game Minecraft and can play it and not go outside. I don't really want to go outside. I just want to stay in my room and play Minecraft, okay? I really am fine with having Asperger's and entomophobia. No big deal. They kind of go together in my mind. Of course, most kids with Asperger's don't have entomophobia, and most kids with entomophobia don't have Asperger's, but I bet a lot have both I will have to look that up. I kind of like having both. I am the bug expert, remember?"

At this point, I discussed with Sam's parents how therapies can be very different and that cognitive behavioral therapy can be particularly effective with phobias. I also expressed how important it was for Sam's parents to be on the same page with each other and with the therapist about his anxiety. Clearly, if they just complied with what Sam wanted, there would be no progress.

Tara and Lenny agreed to meet again to discuss this and not keep things the way they were, even though there was pushback from Sam, . . . and even though Tara had mixed feelings.

"Well, it is clear Sam doesn't want to engage in this treatment," she said. "He wants nothing to do with these goals. He wants to stay at home, in his room playing Minecraft, and doing his own thing away from kids and away from bugs." She hesitated, then continued. "Maybe that's what he should do. Kids with Asperger's like to be alone, right? Should we impose our goals on him if he doesn't want to work on this? He needs to have his voice heard, right? He hated the last therapy. He finally said, 'Mom, why am I seeing that doctor? He knew nothing about Minecraft, and even after I taught him, how is this helping with my bug problem?'"

Tara said she'd had to agree that there had been no progress, so they had stopped therapy, and I could understand her frustration when she wondered if they were now pushing too hard to make him be someone he's not.

"We accept the Asperger's," she continued. "I think we need to accept that this is just part of it and stop pressuring him about it. I don't want him to start feeling bad about himself. He seems happy playing inside. Doesn't he have the right to make a decision about therapy? Since he really wants no part of this, can we drag him in here?"

Lenny sighed, looked at me, and said, "We have a good marriage, but honestly, this is the thing we fight about. I'm sorry, but I think my wife is way too overprotective of Sam. I know he's special, and he has Asperger's, but everyone agrees his Asperger's is mild, and his anxiety is the problem. That's what the school says, and that's what everyone who meets with him says: very smart boy—gifted, in fact—mild Asperger's, severe anxiety. So I think we have to help him with the anxiety. I can't see how letting him avoid situations is the right thing to do. I know that's what he wants. Let's face it, he will never work on his fears unless we push him."

He went on. "And we both have to agree it's the right thing to do. I've done a lot of reading about all this. I think cognitive behavioral therapy is the way to go, and we've never tried it before with Sam. I know he's almost 14 years old, and that's what worries me. We have a small window now to influence him and get him help. I don't want my son to grow up to be a man who's afraid to go outside because of bugs. What kind of life will that be for him? We don't want him living in our basement on the computer."

In a positive way, Lenny confronted Tara, saying that in the past, Sam had always known his mom would give in and let Sam avoid things.

"You're a great mother," Larry said, "but you never agreed on pushing him, so let's face it, we failed. His anxiety has gotten the better of us, and it's gotten worse with time, not better. He's way too comfortable isolating himself and acting different from his peers. I think he can be much more mainstreamed."

Tara shook her head. "I don't think this is fair. We need to hear his voice. If he doesn't want to work on these goals, we shouldn't force him."

Lenny now raised his voice in frustration. "His only hope is to get over this anxiety so he can reach his potential. I understand you don't want us to force him into goals he doesn't agree with, but what exactly are his goals? He wants to stay alone and play computer games. That can't be good for him. I know he said he wants no part of this therapy and says he's fine the way he is. Well, he's not fine. He should be able to go outside. He loves nature. He loves animals. He'd love to pet all those animals at the farm like he used to. Now he can't because of this bug thing. His life has become so limited, not by his Asperger's, but by his fears.

"If it takes incentives, bribes, limits, whatever, we need to get him over this. I think he can do it. He needs to be pushed, and we can push. If we don't help him out of this now, we will only have a bigger problem later."

Tara was still unconvinced and reluctant to force Sam back into therapy to get over his fears. "His mind doesn't work like everyone else's. How is this going to work anyway? What kind of rewards can we give him? He's smart, you know. He'll know we're just bribing him to do this."

Lenny was calmer now and simply said, "I will bribe him. I don't care what he thinks. I just want to be able to go outside and take a walk with my son, ride bikes like we used to, go into the city. Let's face it, this problem is affecting our whole family. Do you think our daughter hasn't noticed that we never do any family activities anymore? What do you think our vacation is going to look like this summer? Even if he goes to a computer camp all summer, I'm not having some kind of indoor computer vacation with my family. I know you may disagree, but this is our son, and our opportunity to help him is now. If we wait, it will be harder."

Tara listened intently and then finally said, "I guess you're right. I just find it hard to impose our values on him since he has Asperger's, and we need to respect that he's different."

"Hey, no one is trying to change the fact that he has some type of autism," Larry said. "But think about it. We're talking about helping him get free from his anxiety. If our daughter had this phobia, would we, for a minute, think we should let her avoid activities and not get over this fear? No. So the same should be for Sam. If we can help him to be less anxious, doesn't he deserve that?"

Thinking about it that way helped Tara to get on board with helping Sam.

It's not unusual for parents to disagree on how much to push their child to fight the anxiety and how much to give in to it. For one thing, giving in to it is easier in the short term. And it can be confusing sorting out how much of this is not anxiety but a feature of something else like Asperger syndrome or being shy or introverted. In the end, Tara and Lenny agreed to help Sam with his anxiety.

We discussed the steps and needed to have an initial discussion about the rewards and incentives first, before we started with Sam. Without powerful incentives that both parents can agree on, we would not even get Sam to the next appointment to start the work. Even though we would discuss the specific rewards and how he would earn them later in the process, Sam needed positive motivation to even get started with the therapy, so exciting him about the idea of earning prizes was needed from the start. Sam was a child who seemed to have everything, and since he was avoiding activities because of his anxiety, we were limited in our choices for rewards. His parents had to start a point system for Sam, and their first homework was to come up with a list of incentives that could motivate him to even come to therapy. They could then offer him points for coming to each meeting, in addition to doing the actual CBT. We also needed to be very positive with Sam about this process. The kids who are the most resistant to this work feel this way because they are so scared to challenge their anxiety; they are afraid it will be too hard.

After convincing Tara, it was time to help Sam realize he could do this . . . step by step.

Step 1: Target Anxious Thoughts and Behaviors

Sam and his parents arrived for their first session together with Sam. "Sam is not happy being here," Lenny said. "It was a struggle to get him to come."

Sam sat down and looked at his hands, where he was fiddling with a toy. He quickly announced, "I am only here for the points. I got fifty points for doing this."

His mother quickly reminded him that if he wanted his points, he also had to cooperate, and he reluctantly agreed. So we started with Sam making a list of his anxious thoughts about bugs:

- They could bite, and that would hurt.
- They feel creepy on my skin.
- The flying thing just scares me.
- They could fly into my mouth or my ear. Yuck, who knows where they could fly into?
- I have never been stung by a bee. What if I'm allergic? I could die!
- What if African killer bees come after me?
- The biggest thing I'm scared of is getting stung. I bet it hurts a lot. I never want to get stung.
- Bugs are interesting, yes, but really very gross.

We then challenged these thoughts. For example:

- Some bugs sting or bite, and it can hurt, but it is not unbearable—it is just a sting. We reminded Sam of how strong he was and how he had broken his finger once, which hurt much more than any bug bite.
- African killer bees are not in our area. They do not kill; they are just more aggressive.
- Bees usually sting us when they feel attacked, as a defense. Their primary interest is not to attack us.
- Bees are important for our food supply and to make honey.
- Bugs that land on our skin, like a fly, don't usually stay for long, and it feels like a tickle more than anything else. As soon as you move or swat the bug, it flies away.
- Bugs can be "gross," but some bugs are beautiful when you look at pictures of them up close.

Then we listed his anxious behaviors:

- Avoidance was primary.
- Not going outside unless absolutely necessary.
- Running to and from the car when I have to go anywhere.
- Not going to the bus stop.
- Not going outside at recess or gym.
- Not being able to look at a bug.
- If there is a fly in the house, screaming and running until someone can catch it and kill it.
- Checking around the house to make sure there are no flying bugs.

Okay, one step at a time.

Step 2: Rate the Anxious Behavior

Again we had to break down Sam's avoidance behaviors into small steps.

Sam was ready to rate 0 to 10. He called 0 "too easy" and 10 "Don't you dare ask me to do this!," which we changed to "Don't you dare ask me to do this *yet!*":

- Walking to and from the car, instead of running in fear **6**
- Not screaming when there is a bug in the house **4**
- Going out the back door and standing outside for five minutes **6**
- Walking with Mom or Dad around the backyard **8**
- Looking at a fly in a jar **6**
- Going to a butterfly garden where butterflies fly around **8**
- Looking at YouTube videos of bugs **2**

It's one thing to rate behaviors, and another thing to agree on dealing with them.

Step 3: Agree on Challenges to Work On

Sam reviewed his list of what to work on:

- Looking at a bug in a jar ("You can't let it get out, right?")
- Not screaming when a bug is in the house
- Walking to and from the car without running
- Looking at YouTube videos of bugs
- Going out the back door and standing outside for five minutes

We all agreed that these were baby steps toward helping Sam feel less anxious about bugs and more able to be outside. Once he realized we weren't going to make him do something that was too scary and that he had control over what was expected of him, he became less resistant and more cooperative. Many kids are resistant because they don't want to feel that horrible panicky feeling and think that's what we are going to make them do. Understanding that he needed to challenge his anxiety but not be overwhelmed by it helped Sam feel like this could work.

We had to start where he was comfortable and build from there, and this seemed promising.

Step 4: Initiate and Teach Strategies to Practice

Sam agreed to write down and then read his challenges to his anxious thoughts. For instance:

- He learned "self-talk," where he reminded himself of what was real and that he was not in danger from bugs.
- He learned to pay attention to his breathing in the fresh air and to the pleasant smells, sights, and feelings of being outside. He needed to remember what he used to like so much about being outside and about nature, instead of hyperfocusing on bugs and reacting with fear.

We then did some focused relaxation exercises. Sam closed his eyes and focused on his breathing being slow and deep, in and out. I then guided him to imagine being outside, helping him focus on positive smells and sounds of the outdoors: the birds singing, the sound of the wind, the feeling of the cool air on his face. I helped him to think of a time when he had fun and enjoyed being outside and to remember what that felt like. He agreed to practice that at home.

We also did *imaginal exposures*, where I guided him to imagine being outside with bugs. Imaginal exposures can be a useful step in desensitizing a child when a real exposure may not be possible or is, at that point, too difficult. They can be a good first step.

Sam, becoming more engaged, closed his eyes, did his breathing, imagined being outside when everything was pleasant, and then added bugs to the picture. He was hearing the bugs, seeing the bugs, feeling the bugs, and looking at the bugs without fear—noticing the bugs rather than reacting to them. This was far more difficult for him to do, but with practice, he became better able to stay calm and keep his breathing even as he visualized being around flying insects. He also practiced this at home.

Step 5: Note and Chart Progress Made

Together, the family designed Sam's chart. Sam happened to be a great artist and got excited about drawing pictures of flying bugs all over his chart.

Step 6: Offer Incentives to Motivate

With Sam, this was the first step, just to get him to agree to work with us. So he continued to get points for coming to the therapy sessions but most important, he also earns points for doing the work he agreed on. What will he get for his points?

His parents had discussed this in advance with Sam and come up with this list:

- Gift certificate to bookstore
- iTunes gift card
- App for his iPad
- Extra time on the weekends for use of computer
- Choosing where the family will get takeout on Friday nights

- Staying up a half hour later on Friday or Saturday night
- New computer game

At this point, Sam's parents raised an important issue. Sam had a sister who was just two years younger. Allison already felt jealous of the attention Sam got. Tara asked, "What is Allison going to feel when she sees Sam getting these rewards for doing what she does every day? I bet she's going to feel angry about all this, or worse, feel like she has to have fears to get rewards. How do we handle that?"

This was a good question and is a common issue when there are siblings. The best option was to talk with Allison about what she could work on. This would help Sam to realize that everyone has something to work on; he's not the "problem child." And it helps Allison to share in getting positive reinforcement for working on her challenges.

It was agreed that Allison would get points for doing things that were hard for her. She had a hard time making her bed and cleaning up after herself, and she easily raised her voice with her parents. She made her own chart and was happy to be earning prizes too.

Step 7: Reinforce Progress and Increase Challenges

After three weeks, Sam came back to my office with his parents, and his mood was certainly much better than at our last meeting. He was smiling and glad to show off his chart and his progress.

We looked at his chart:

- Now walking to and from the car was **0**, so we crossed that off the list.
- After standing outside in the backyard, he was now able to sit outside on the deck. His parents had the idea of bringing a board game out there that he could play with his sister. He had been out there over two hours and said it was a **0** if there were no bugs, a **5** if he saw a bug flying around.
- Relaxation and imaginal exposures were now easy: **0**.
- Looking at the YouTube videos, easy: **0**.
- Not screaming if a fly is in the house couldn't be worked on because no fly had come into the house: **5**.
- Looking at a fly in a jar, easy: **0**.

Now Sam was ready for the next steps.

- He agreed to walk around the block with his mom or dad. 7
- He would continue to work on being in the backyard on the deck. 5
- He agreed to shoot baskets in the driveway. 7
- He agreed to go out for recess. **Rating 5.** The longer he stays out and doesn't come in the school, the more points he earns. We discussed what he could do outside, and his mom agreed to call his school to make sure he can be helped to join a group outside so he's not alone out there worrying about bugs.

At one session, Sam's sister, Allison, joined us and showed off her chart. She was working on making her bed and keeping her room clean, not leaving her dishes in the family room, keeping her voice down, and not screaming when she got upset. She had also earned points for a gift certificate at the bookstore and was working on points for a trip to the mall with her mom.

Next Steps

Sam was on his way, and although the progress had been slow, it was tangible, and Sam was proud of himself, despite all the original protestations.

Both his parents agreed to get a medication consultation to help Sam overcome his fears. Since starting on his medication, he has been less anxious and more able to move up his goals. We continue to meet monthly, and he has been able to go on a walk with his father for fifteen minutes. Next, he plans on visiting a local farm and petting the animals.

* * *

Both Ellen and Sam experienced anxiety in different ways, and their parents had different opinions on how to respond. Parents can be enablers of anxiety, especially when children seem very comfortable in their avoidance. Parents understandably want to avoid a struggle with their child. Many anxious children are very resistant to change, and although they are often not functioning up to their potential, they are still functioning.

Parents often experience conflicts about how to deal with an anxious child. Resolving these conflicts and getting parents to work together can be an important part of this process.

DSM-5 Guidelines

Specific Phobia

The *DSM-5* identifies the diagnostic criteria necessary for a diagnosis. The assumption is that many readers will have children who meet some but not all the criteria.

A. Marked fear or anxiety about a specific object or situation (e.g., flying, heights, animals, receiving an injection, seeing blood).

> Note: In children, the fear or anxiety may be expressed by crying, tantrums, freezing, or clinging.

B. The phobic object or situation almost always provokes immediate fear or anxiety.

C. The phobic object or situation is actively avoided or endured with intense fear or anxiety.

D. The fear or anxiety is out of proportion to the actual danger posed by the specific object or situation and to the sociocultural context.

E. The fear, anxiety, or avoidance is persistent, typically lasting for six months or more.

F. The fear, anxiety, or avoidance causes clinically significant distress or impairment in social, occupational, or other important areas of functioning.

G. The disturbance is not better explained by the symptoms of another mental disorder, including fear, anxiety, and avoidance of situations associated with panic-like symptoms or other incapacitating symptoms (as in agoraphobia); objects or situations related to obsessions (as in obsessive-compulsive disorder); reminders of traumatic events (as in post-traumatic stress disorder); separation from home or attachment figures (as in separation anxiety disorder).

Specify if:

Code based on the phobic stimulus:

300.29 (F40.218) Animal (e.g., spiders, insects, dogs).

300.29 (F40.228) Natural environment (e.g., heights, storms, water).

300.29 (F40.23x) Blood-injection-injury (e.g., needles, invasive medical procedures).

> **Coding note:** Select specific ICD-10-CM code as follows: **F40.230** fear of blood; **F40.231** fear of injections and transfusions; **F40.232** fear of other medical care; or **F40.233** fear of injury.

300.29 (F40.248) Situational (e.g., airplanes, elevators, enclosed places).

300.29 (F40.298) Other (e.g., situations that may lead to choking or vomiting; in children, e.g., loud sounds or costumed characters).

> **Coding note:** When more than one phobic stimulus is present, code all ICD-10-CM codes that apply (e.g., for fear of snakes and flying, F40.218 specific phobia, animal, and F40.248 specific phobia, situational).

American Psychiatric Association. "Specific Phobia." In *Diagnostic and Statistical Manual of Mental Disorders*. 5th ed. Washington, DC: American Psychiatric Association, 2013.

Chapter 8

When Bad Things Happen to Good Kids

Post-Traumatic Stress Disorder

Post-traumatic stress disorder (PTSD) is an anxiety disorder that is triggered by a terrifying event—directly experiencing it or witnessing it. The symptoms include intrusive memories of the event; the feeling of re-experiencing it (flashbacks); avoiding situations that are associated with the event; feeling numb or without feelings, especially right after the event; becoming hypervigilant, which can include being irritable; having trouble concentrating and sleeping; always being "on guard" due to a fear of being in danger; and becoming easily startled.

Young children with PTSD may experience more separation anxiety and have more trouble with toilet training, going to the bathroom, or bedwetting. Older children may act out the trauma through play, drawings, or stories. They may have more physical complaints and become more fearful and anxious. This anxiety could be expressed through avoidance, or aggressive behavior, or both.

Complex PTSD develops after the experience of prolonged trauma. Combat veterans and people who experienced child abuse have suffered many traumatic experiences. With multiple experiences of traumatic events, the treatment usually involves a multimodal approach, in which cognitive behavioral therapy (CBT) can be part of the treatment but is not the only approach. CBT can be most effective alone when the person has experienced only a single traumatic event.

This chapter walks you through two representative stories of children who have PTSD.

John and Carolyn's Story

These parents were distraught when they saw me about their daughter, 3½-year-old Molly.

Carolyn started the session: "Eight months ago, we were eating in a restaurant, and the waitress was pouring my tea and someone bumped into her from behind, and the waitress poured boiling hot water on Molly's shoulder and down her arm. It was horrible. Molly screamed. The waitress screamed. I screamed. It was chaos."

Carolyn started to cry and couldn't talk.

John jumped in. "I grabbed her out of her high chair and ripped her clothes off her as quickly as I could. She screamed so loudly. Someone called 911, and an ambulance came with the sirens and the lights, and she was rushed to the hospital. It was a nightmare; she was so hurt and scared. We were with her but couldn't hold her because of the burns. It was by far the worst day of my life. Since then, she's been back and forth to doctors, and amazingly, it's healed. Of course she has scars, and I'm not sure if they'll ever go away. But thank God, the pain is gone. We had to keep bandages on and change the bandages frequently to avoid infection. It never got infected. The doctors say she's now pain-free. But I know it must've hurt her so much."

Carolyn then spoke. "Our problem now is she's afraid of water. I mean any water that gets on her body. Giving her a bath is impossible. She screams like she's being burned all over again. I can't bear it. It brings it all back for me, seeing her looking so scared. So we take a cloth with soap and water and gently clean her. We know this can't go on. She has to get over this."

"Honestly, John added, "we thought this would all just go away with time. We hoped she would forget what happened, and she's so little. But her fear of water is not going away, so she must still be haunted. We know she has to be able to take a bath. We just don't know what to do. Now that summer's coming, we were hoping we could get her in a pool or go to the beach with her. That seems impossible now. We don't know how to help her."

I explained that I've seen other young and old people undergo similar traumas. We could deal with it methodically.

Step 1: Target Anxious Thoughts and Behaviors

Molly was so little, and she had experienced a significant trauma. Because of how young she is, she can't understand how to put this horrible burn in perspective. Her anxious thought is "Water will hurt me." Her anxious behavior is to avoid any water, and when she gets near water, to scream in fear as if she's about to be burned all over again.

So we needed to start with changing her thoughts and feelings about water. She would benefit most from graduated exposure to water to help her overcome her fear.

Step 2: Rate the Anxious Thoughts and Behavior

I suggested we start with a water table for her to play with water inside. Because she was so little, her parents provided the ratings based on their experiences with her.

- Standing at the water table and playing with toys in a little bit of water   **5**
- At the water table, putting a little water on her arm and shoulder where she had been burned   **10**
- Standing in a kiddie pool with water in it   **5**
- Sitting in a kiddie pool with water   **8**
- Standing in the tub   **8**
- Sitting in the tub with water   **10**
- Sitting in the tub playing, with no water   **6**
- Singing with parents and with music, sitting in the tub with toys and a little water   **8**
- Going to the pool and watching other kids playing in the water   **7**
- Putting her feet in the water at the pool   **8**

I suggested that they avoid touching her burn area with water since that triggers her to scream right away. She needed to feel more comfortable with water and build up to putting water where she was burned. That would be the last step. The parents agreed, and we went on to the next step.

Step 3: Agree on Challenges to Work On

Carolyn said, "I know this all makes sense. We have to gradually help her get used to water. But honestly, I get so nervous even thinking about this. I don't want her to be hurt and scared anymore, yet I wish she didn't have to go through all this."

I explained that if they weren't comfortable doing this with her, she would pick up on their anxiety and become more afraid. We could take small steps in exposing her to water, I said. We didn't want to overwhelm and retraumatize her. She would feel scared and uncomfortable at the start of each step, but then she would relax.

I stressed that they had to be willing not only to tolerate her discomfort, but to stay composed, and when she was afraid, to guide her through it. They needed to make it playful and be lighthearted with her to help her experience that water is not going to hurt her. It can instead be fun.

"You need to know," John said, "that my wife, I think, blames herself for all this. She thinks somehow it's her fault. She says things like 'I shouldn't have put the high chair there. I shouldn't have ordered tea, and we should have had dinner at home.' Some nights she goes on and on like this. No matter what I say, it doesn't seem to help."

We then turned the conversation away from Molly, and they spoke about what all this has been like for them. Carolyn said, "You're right, that's how I think sometimes, and I can't help it. It's been hard. I had nightmares. They've gotten better, but at first, I couldn't sleep at all. I kept dreaming Molly was suffering in all kinds of horrific ways, and I couldn't get to her. I couldn't save her. Every night, I dreaded going to sleep."

John put his arm around her. "For weeks after this happened," he said, "she'd wake up crying, and Molly would be crying. None of us got any sleep. I felt like I couldn't do enough to help them. I also still feel guilty, especially when I look at her scars. I'm her dad. It's my job to protect her. It's hard not to feel like I failed in some major way."

We talked about how, by witnessing this, they too were traumatized. If they didn't lessen their own anxiety, it would be hard for them to help Molly relax and recover from her experience. They agreed to see a couples' therapist who specializes in PTSD to help them recover as a couple from this trauma.

John felt strongly that he was able to start the exposure therapy with Molly. "I really think I can do this, and it will help me feel like I'm doing something to help her. So far I've felt helpless, not knowing what to do for her. We really have fun together. I love playing with her, and she easily laughs with me. I want to get started with this."

Carolyn looked relieved, knowing she wasn't ready to experience Molly's discomfort. Avoiding water with Molly, and trying to forget it ever happened, was her way of coping.

We all agreed that standing in a kiddie pool in the family room, where Molly loves to play, was the best way to start. She and her dad love to dance together in the family room with music, so putting on the music and dancing with Dad in the pool with a little water sounded like a good first step. We also thought putting new water toys in the pool might get her curious enough to want to play in the water. In addition to that, they agreed to set up a water table with new toys so Molly could stand and put her hands in the water to play with the toys.

We were on our way.

Step 4: Initiate and Teach Strategies to Practice

We agreed to the following strategies:

- Keep everything playful.
- Use music and laughter and keep her playing through the exposures.
- Talk to Molly over and over again about how great water is, to help her change the way she thinks.
- Use every opportunity to model what fun water can be. Let her see you having fun with water.
- Keep relaxed and confident. Remember you are guiding her through her fear of water. She needs to feel from you that she's safe doing this.
- Since she loves bubbles, have her blow them when she's anxious. This will help with her breathing.

Overall, we decided to go slowly with each step, being patient and following Molly's lead, since I expected that Molly would let them know when she was relaxed and ready for the next step. I reminded the parents not to overwhelm her by pushing her too fast.

Step 5: Note and Chart Progress Made

Though Molly can't rate her progress, her parents can based on her reaction to the exposures. John was confident that he could measure her discomfort based on observing her, and they would keep a chart with a simple rating of easy, hard, very hard, and couldn't do it. It was very important that they stay in the easy-to-hard range. She shouldn't become overwhelmed by the exposure; it shouldn't be too anxiety producing for her. We wanted it to be challenging but not overwhelming and as positive as possible. It's most important to be playful in this process, even if that takes longer to make progress.

Step 6: Offer Incentives to Motivate

As is often the case, positive reinforcement will be very important to make this work. Molly loves stickers and M&Ms, so that's what we went for.

Carolyn said, "It worked like a charm for toilet training. I bet it'll work for this too." Her parents would take her out to choose stickers and explain that she can get stickers and candy for playing the "water game" with Daddy. Her parents thought she would be very excited about this. She was really in love with princesses, so princess stickers would be great. I encouraged them to use a big sticker for when she did something new that she hadn't yet done with water, and smaller ones for practicing the same water activity. Similarly, they should give her more M&Ms for the first time she took a new step in increasing her exposure to water. The first time is always the hardest, and then it gets easier.

Step 7: Reinforce Progress and Increase Challenges

After a month, we met and discussed Molly's progress.

Carolyn started. "First I want to tell you, John and I have been seeing another therapist to help us with this. It's helped me realize how intense my feelings about all this are. I'm working on it, and even started working a little with John on the exposures with Molly. The exposures are really helping her feel less afraid."

John described what had been going on. "We started with the water table and standing in the pool. It was tough at first to get her to do it. But I kept being patient and offering more and more candy. Finally, she took the bait and went in. She looked scared, but I got her laughing and singing. We kept doing it, and she gradually became more relaxed. I couldn't figure out how to get her to sit in the water and play. I know this sounds ridiculous, and it sure looks ridiculous, but we bought a big kiddie pool, big enough for me to get in. I set it up in the family room, got in my bathing suit, filled the pool with some water and all her water toys, and I started playing in the pool. It was big enough for both of us to sit in it. She watched me and before long put one foot in, and then the next, and ended up sitting with me in the water playing."

Carolyn said, "When I saw that, I started to laugh and cry. Looking at my husband in that ridiculous pool, and seeing her sitting and playing in the water, it made me feel so happy. I know she's getting better."

Now it was time to talk about next goals:

- Taking a bath. Transferring her from the pool to the tub would be a challenge. We discussed first bathing her with fun bubbles in the pool and then gradually getting her in the tub with her dad.
- Going swimming in a real pool. We discussed taking her to the YMCA pool, where she could first watch kids play in the water, then gradually put her feet in the water, with Dad close to her. Next, Dad would play in the water while Mom stayed with her on the side, watching until she was ready for Dad to place her in the water. This would be a huge accomplishment and would probably take many visits to the pool.
- Exposing her burn area to water. Molly would still get scared and start to cry if any water touched the skin where she was burned. Doctors had reassured her parents that the burn was healed and that it no longer hurt her. It was her fear that was now causing her pain. We discussed gradually having drops of water fall on that area when she was in the kiddie pool and rewarding her right away, reinforce over and over that water would not hurt her. They would continue doing this, slowly having more and more water touch her burn area.

Through these exposures, Molly was starting to experience water as something fun. She was changing the way she felt about water and how she acted with water.

Carolyn said, "It's really working now. Before we learned how to do this, we were pushing her too hard to get into the water. Our goals were too high, and she couldn't do it. Then we created this cycle where she would get anxious and start screaming, and I would overreact, as if she was in pain, and quickly get her away from the water. We'd both be a mess after that and give up. We were stuck. If anything, that probably gave her the message again and again that water is dangerous."

Carolyn and John have since learned how graduated exposure works; they have also learned how they had to heal along with Molly to recover from the trauma they all experienced when she was burned.

We continued to meet monthly, and after seven months, Molly was doing really well in the water. Her fear had greatly diminished. Carolyn and John made good use of their couples' therapy, which helped them realize how traumatized they had been by experiencing Molly getting burned. They were healing as a family from the burn, which was not just physical but psychological for the whole family.

Next Steps

It took several months of just about daily water play, but Molly made consistent progress and is now able to go in the pool with her parents. Meanwhile, Carolyn and John have continued in their therapy and are working on healing their own PTSD. One of the things they realized in therapy was that deep down, not only did they blame themselves for what happened, they blamed each other. They had known they were often angry at each other since the accident, but they hadn't realized why. The more they accepted that they were not to blame for what happened to Molly, the better they felt. Unexpectedly to them, this process helped strengthen their marriage.

Maura and John's Story

Maura and John came to see me because they were worried about their 19-year-old daughter, Monica. As is usually my approach, I let the parents ventilate without interrupting.

Maura started. "Monica just finished her freshman year at college. She was always a happy kid. We never had any problems with her, beyond the usual stuff. In high school she had a busy social life but kept her grades up and worked hard. She got into her first choice school. It's a large university. We thought she might do better in a smaller school, but she wanted large.

"She always had lots of good friends," she continued. "I guess you could say she was popular. As far as I know, she drank a little at parties her senior year, and I imagine she smoked pot. She never had any problems with that stuff though. Twice she was late for curfew in her senior year, and we grounded her, and that was it. She usually respected our rules."

John looked impatient and interrupted. "The reason we're here is that she's coming home from school for the summer, and she told us she needs to see a therapist."

Maura continued. "I'm sorry. I didn't mean to get off track, but I wanted you to know a little about her. Anyway, John's right, she needs to see a doctor to talk to. She won't tell us why. That's the hard part. If only we knew, maybe we could help her. I'm worried sick. I know something's wrong. I just don't know what it is."

Nervously, Maura went on, "She had a great first semester at school. She was home at Thanksgiving and Christmas and seemed really happy. Her grades were great too. All A's except one B in math. She was making friends, had good roommates. Everything seemed fine. When she came home for March break, something had changed. She seemed . . . reserved, quiet, no emotions. I don't know how to explain it. Low energy, in her room, sleeping a lot, not herself, but every time I'd ask her, she'd say she's fine. She didn't want to see her high school friends, which was a big red flag for me.

"At night, sometimes, I could hear her crying in her room. We were always so close; she used to tell me everything. If she had a problem, she always came to me. I asked her older sister to talk to her and Monica said the same thing to her—everything's fine.

"Well, Monica went back to school after the break, and every time I'd talk to her, she seemed down, irritable, like I was bothering her by calling. At first I felt hurt, since she never acted like this toward me before. I wondered if I did something to upset her. So I backed off and stopped calling her so much. But she called me crying last night. Her semester is over, and she's coming home in a week. Her grades are down, all Cs and one B. I don't care about that, but she said she's not sleeping, and she's having panic attacks. She never had this problem before. Maybe this school is not right for her? I don't know . . ."

Maura became tearful. "I just wish I knew what was wrong and how to help her."

John took up the conversation. "She was always a happy kid. I don't get it. I hope she didn't take drugs or something like that. Could that cause this? I just keep imagining the worst. I don't know what got her in this state. But we have to decide if she should go back to school, or maybe she needs some time off. I always thought she shouldn't be so far away from home in such a large school. Maybe it's just too much for her. She's sensitive, you know."

John paused. "She's supposed to work this summer as a lifeguard. She's had that job for three years. I hope she can do it. Can you help us figure this out? Can you help her?"

It was clear that I needed to meet with Monica, and the fact that she had expressed needing to talk to a therapist was a good sign. So we arranged for her to see me without her parents.

Monica's Story

Monica came in looking scared and was hesitant at first. "I don't know how to do this. I've never gone to a therapist before. I just know I need help, and I promised my roommate I would get help over the summer." She then started to cry. "I'm sorry . . . I don't know where to begin."

I told her that she was in a safe place and that she could start by telling me what had brought her here. She regained her composure and continued: "I'm having trouble sleeping. I have nightmares. And sometimes I get panic attacks, like my heart is beating so fast, and I feel like I can't breathe, and I get hot and sweaty. I also sometimes can't concentrate. My grades have gone down this semester. I don't know how I got through it. I'm glad I'm home, and I thought being home would help, but I have the same feelings."

I asked her when this all started. "It was several months ago. Something happened to me. I can't really talk about it. I get too upset."

She stopped short and asked, "This is confidential, right? You're not going to tell my parents, are you?"

I reassured her that I would not. I reviewed with her that I would tell her parents only if I thought she was in danger of hurting herself or others.

"No, I'm not suicidal. It's nothing like that," she said.

I asked her to try to tell me what had happened since I couldn't really help without knowing the facts.

She again started to cry and said, "I'm too ashamed."

I explained that talking about it could help with those feelings, and she finally started to open up.

"I was at a frat party, and I was . . ." Her voice trailed to barely a whisper. "Raped. I can't tell my parents. They couldn't handle it. My dad, I swear he would try to track down and kill the guy. I'm serious. They can never find out. They would never let me go back to college. My mom would create a big scene at school. She'd want to sue them or something. She's a lawyer. They would be so disappointed in me. I don't want them to ever find out. I'm close to my mother, but she can never know this happened to me. I just want to stop feeling these feelings and be back to myself. I know I need help to get over this. I thought it would just go away, but it's not. I wish I could just forget about it."

I assured Monica that she wasn't alone and that I was confident our strategic approach would help her feel better.

Step 1: Target the Anxious Thoughts and Behaviors

It was hard for Monica to describe her thoughts, but it was time to get to work, and Monica tried to cooperate: "Most of the time I'm fine, but sometimes, I feel panic come over me, like I can't breathe. I feel like something bad is going to happen. I get even a bit paranoid. Like someone's going to jump out of nowhere and hurt me. Sometimes, while studying in my room, my roommate would walk in, and I would jump like a bolt of lightning."

She took in a deep breath and forged ahead. "I feel like I can't trust guys anymore. I'm sometimes afraid of them. I feel angry at myself now. How could I have let this happen to me? Sometimes I think I'm bad or dirty in some way. I know I'm not. It wasn't my fault, but it feels like I should have prevented it. It's confusing."

I asked Monica to elaborate.

"I have nightmares over and over again, the same kind of dreams. I'm always helpless, and bad things, violent things are happening to me and I can't stop it, until I wake up crying and in a sweat. It feels so real. I wake up, and I feel exhausted."

I explained to Monica that she had post-traumatic stress disorder (PTSD), which was common after being raped. I encouraged her to learn more about PTSD.

She said, "No, I'm sorry. Usually I like to learn about things, but when it comes to this, I don't want to read about it. I just want it all to go away. My goal is just to forget about it and move on."

Concluding this first session, I told her that to understand her anxious thoughts more clearly, she needed to learn more about rape and the common feelings victims feel after being raped. This would help her feel less alone. I stressed that what she's experiencing is a normal reaction to what happened to her and that talking about it with me would help her feel better and then be more able to feel relaxed and less anxious.

She came into the next session ready to tell me what had happened that night. I explained to her that we could do it at her own pace; she could take breaks if necessary. I reminded her that this should be challenging but not overwhelming. Certainly, I didn't want her to be retraumatized by becoming flooded with uncomfortable feelings. She was confident that she could tell me, since she had told several of her friends already. She also said, "I already told my doctor and have been tested for sexually transmitted diseases, which, thank God, were all negative."

Then she began to describe what had happened. "It was a Friday night, in the second week of February. I had stayed up half the night before, studying for a test, and I was tired. My roommate, Stacey, told me about this frat party. I was tired and didn't really feel like going out, but she convinced me that it could be fun. I told her I probably would want to leave early, and she was fine with that. Stacey and I had become good friends, and she's a lot of fun to go out with, but I can't help but think I should have listened to my gut and not gone. If I didn't go to that stupid party, none of this would've happened to me. I keep thinking of that. Anyway, we went to the party. I had a few beers. I know how to drink. I drank in high school, got trashed a few times, and don't like that feeling."

I told her she was doing great and asked her to continue. "I don't drink a lot; everybody here knows that about me. I didn't even smoke weed that night. I knew that would put me right to sleep, because I was so tired to begin with. So, we had been there for a few hours, the music and so many people made it very loud. I was ready to go back to the dorm and went to find Stacey, because we'd agreed to walk back together. We felt safer that way. Ironic, isn't it? We thought it was dangerous to walk alone at night, and I get raped at a big party, with lots of people around. It makes no sense. So I was walking around looking for her, and I heard my name called."

At this point Monica slowed down. "This is where it all went bad. It was Don. He's a junior, pre-med. We'd hung out a little in the fall. I hadn't seen or heard from him in months. I figured I'd talk to him for a few minutes. He said something like he wanted to catch up with me. I went into this room with him and quickly realized he was drunk. Really drunk. He smelled like hard liquor, weed, and sweat, all combined. I remember thinking I was too tired to listen to him slur his words and talk nonsense, I just wanted to go back to my dorm, to sleep. But I didn't want to be rude. How stupid is that? Why was I worrying about being rude? I should have just left right then. I quickly told him I was tired and heading back to my dorm.

"He said, 'Oh no, you're not.'

"I thought he was kidding, and I said, 'Oh yes, I am. Stacey's waiting downstairs for me.'

"At that point he grabbed me hard and pulled me down. I remember telling him to stop, to leave me alone; I still couldn't believe what he was doing. I told him he was hurting me and tried to get away. Then, I will never forget this, he said, 'Shut up, bitch.'

"I started to struggle, and he put his hands around my neck like he was going to strangle me. Then I was really scared. That's when time seemed to slow down. I felt like I was going to die. I never felt that before."

Tears started to roll down Monica's face. She was shaking, and her face and neck were beet red. I suggested she might want to take a break. She said, "No, I'm fine. I know it's over. I really thought I could die. He's a big guy, a football player. I don't know why I didn't scream. Or bite him or punch him. Why didn't I fight more? If I fought more, maybe this wouldn't have happened. I got so scared, I froze. I remember him being so big, on top of me, hurting me and out of control. And then, it was over, just like that. He got up, and this is weird, he mumbled something about it being good, and stumbled out of the room, leaving me there. I got up and felt . . . nothing, numb, like I was in a daze.

"I guess I was just walking around, and Stacey came up to me. She knew immediately something was wrong. She asked if I was okay. I told her I just needed to get out of there. We left and started walking back to the dorm. Right away, she asked me about my neck. She said it was all red. She kept asking me what was wrong. I didn't want to tell her. I didn't know what to say, I felt so ashamed. How could I have let this happen to me? Finally, I blurted out, 'I was just raped.'

"I remember the words coming out of my mouth with no emotion. I felt nothing, nothing except dirty. I felt filthy dirty. I just wanted to take a shower and wash all this off me. Stacey was shocked and so upset, she started to cry. I told her I was fine. I remember she said something about how I should report it. I told her no way. I was not going to report it. I have seen what happens to girls who report these things. It gets ugly. At that point I just wanted to get clean and forget it ever happened.

"As soon as we got to the dorm, I headed straight for the shower and kept washing and washing. I wanted to scrub every inch of my body. I washed until I was too exhausted to continue and had to stop. I still felt dirty. Finally I came back to the room, and Stacey was still up. She asked me who it was. I didn't want to tell her, but then she said, 'Was it Don?' I was surprised and asked her how she knew. She said she heard rumors that he was known to be a creep like this when he was drunk. She said, 'I never believed the stories. He's such a nice guy and so smart, pre-med. He's always talking about going to Harvard where his dad went.' I made her promise not to tell anyone. It was all so confusing. I felt so ashamed. That night, Stacey cried, but I didn't cry. I still felt nothing, numb."

Monica looked at me at this point and asked, "You're not going to tell anyone, are you? Don't make me tell anyone. I don't want to report this to anyone at school. I can't go through that. I know I can't."

I reassured her about confidentiality and that reporting it or not was in her control. Monica started crying. I told her it was good for her to cry, and I asked her to let herself feel what Stacey felt for her that night—so sad that something like this had happened to her.

In the next session, we were ready to take a closer look at her anxious thoughts:

- It was my fault this happened.
- I should've fought harder.
- I could've stopped him.
- I should've screamed and caused a scene.
- I was a complete coward.
- If I hadn't talked to him, this never would have happened. I knew he was wasted; I shouldn't have talked to him.
- If I hadn't gone to this party, it wouldn't have happened. I shouldn't have gone.
- I shouldn't have gone upstairs in that house; I should have kept close to Stacey.
- Maybe it was what I was wearing. I threw out the jeans and sweater I wore that night.

- This could have been prevented. It's my fault this happened.
- I can't let anyone find out about this. They'll think it was my fault and that I'm an idiot. Why did this happen to me? There must be a reason this happened to me and not all the other girls at that party.
- Don isn't a bad person. Everyone thinks he's great. He's on the football team. He's smart. How could he be a rapist? No one would believe he did this to me.
- Now I'm afraid of men. I guess I think any guy could just rape me. I'm scared this will happen again.

Next we worked on challenging those thoughts with facts. I explained to Monica that one in five college girls is sexually assaulted while in college. She was hardly alone. It is an epidemic on campuses across the country. She was shocked to hear that. I told her this was not her fault, but when bad things happen to good people, they tend to blame themselves. Rape victims almost always first blame themselves. I emphasized that she did nothing to cause this to happen, and she couldn't have stopped it. She did what her instincts told her to do, and she was probably right. If she had fought him more, he could have escalated his violence. She was afraid for her life, but she survived his attack, even though she had thought he was going to kill her. He's the criminal who raped her.

As I said these words, tears came streaming down her face. She said, "I never thought of it like that. I don't know why. He's hurt me so much by doing this to me; my whole life has changed since that night. I hate him."

From this point on, we started to see a transformation. Changing how she thought was changing her feelings from numb to sad and even angry. She was starting to challenge her thoughts. We were making progress.

I asked Monica to list her anxious behaviors:

- I get anxious going to parties, especially large parties. I panic.
- I feel like my libido is gone. I avoid guys completely, even the nice ones. I'm afraid of them.
- Oh, the smell of hard liquor and weed, that combination, I can't stand it. It literally makes me sick, and I have to get away. Let's face it, I live on a college campus—that smell is everywhere. But I stay away from it as much as I can.
- I hate walking near where it happened, that frat house.

- I feel ashamed when I talk about it. Like it's my fault.
- I love my parents, and I know they're upset about me and want to know what's wrong, but I can't tell them. I feel too ashamed. I just want to block it all out. I feel like they will think differently about me.

After listing these behaviors, it was time to rate them.

Step 2: Rate the Anxious Thoughts and Behavior

Although Monica felt a high level of anxiety related to the incident, I told her we needed to view the relative numbers before we started to deal with the specific issues.

Her list:

- Going to a small party with friends **3**
- Going to a large party **6**
- Doing anything sexual, including masturbation **7**
- Talking about the details of what happened and not feeling ashamed **8**
- Reading or watching anything about rape or PTSD **3**
- Smelling hard liquor or marijuana **5**
- Telling parents **7**
- Going to frat house **7**
- Walking by frat house and looking at it **4**

This gave us a framework for the next step.

Step 3: Agree on Challenges to Work On

After Monica agreed to write out her anxious, irrational thoughts about being raped, she then needed to write the realistic thoughts. This is called *cognitive restructuring*, helping her change the way she thinks about this trauma. She decided to write it in her phone, so she could read it anytime she found herself feeling bad about herself because of being raped. She wrote: "I was raped. Rape is a crime, and it was not my fault. I'm angry he did this to me. I'm not alone. Too many students are raped, and he probably did this to other students. I shouldn't feel ashamed. I did nothing wrong. I did the best I could. I'm not dirty because of this. All men are not rapists. It's okay to have feelings that are all mixed up. I will feel better." She agreed to read this every day.

This was the cognitive part of the therapy, changing the way she thinks.

She also agreed to do graduated exposures around the things she was avoiding, starting with spending time having fun with her high school friends, who were also home for the summer. She also agreed to read more about rape and learn about how her experience is very typical of victims of rape. She had resisted this because she wanted to avoid anything about rape; she just wanted to forget about it. But she was starting to understand that trying not to think about it only made her anxiety worse. Learning more about rape could only help her change the negative way she was thinking about herself.

It was time to move forward.

Step 4: Initiate and Teach Strategies to Practice

We discussed various relaxation strategies that she could work on. She agreed to learn meditation and practice it twice a day. She also agreed to take a yoga class and practice stretching with deep breathing. Being traumatized often creates an intense physical reaction that can become associated with anxiety, and combining physical relaxation with cognitive restructuring and exposure therapy can be useful in the recovery from trauma.

Monica has felt both numb and flooded with intense feelings. These strategies could help her modulate her feelings and reduce her anxiety. She went back to working as a lifeguard but was worried about having a panic attack at work. It's very common to get anxious after having a panic attack—panicking about panicking. We reviewed what she could do if she had a panic attack. She chose to make a plan for herself that included self-talk (it's just anxiety, it will pass, I'm okay), distraction (go in the pool or take a break and go to the bathroom), and focusing on "grounding herself" (letting all her senses tune in to where she is, so she's in the here and now and not focused on her anxious feelings). She learned to acknowledge her feelings as they moved through her. We practiced this in the office.

Step 5: Note and Chart Progress Made

Monica decided to keep her progress chart in her phone. When she went to chart her progress, she agreed to also read what she had written to challenge her anxious thoughts. She would also keep track of how often she did the following and rate how hard it felt:

- Spending time with guy friends
- Going to parties
- Reading about rape and PTSD

Step 6: Offer Incentives to Motivate

Sometimes, this is the most critical step. Given Monica's age and her strong motivation to feel better, at first glance this step may not seem necessary. In discussing this with Monica, however, we talked about how hard the work was and how she needed to move forward, not backward. She also needed to acknowledge her strength and power as she regained control over her feelings and worked to recover.

She felt ashamed of what happened, so she needed to develop more feelings of pride in her accomplishment as a trauma survivor. She decided to think of ways she could treat herself as she moved along in her goals. She made a list of things she could reward herself with:

- Getting a manicure and pedicure
- Getting a massage
- Getting a frozen yogurt
- Watching a marathon session of the latest TV show she wants to catch up on
- Buying herself a new outfit

Step 7: Reinforce Progress and Increase Challenges

Monica worked hard and was feeling better. She was enjoying yoga and meditation, and she'd been spending more time with friends; she had even gone to two small parties.

We discussed increasing the goals. Even though it was the middle of her summer break, she needed to go back to school for a long weekend to meet with one of her professors, so we discussed doing exposures on campus. She agreed to go to the frat house where it had happened, even just walking by it at first, until that felt okay, and then going inside if she could.

We also discussed her parents, who were still not aware of what had happened. I disclosed to Monica that they had called me. They were concerned about her, and still very worried and confused. They wondered if she should go back to school in September. Monica said again that she felt too ashamed to tell them. We discussed how she would feel about telling them if she had been mugged on campus and her wallet had been stolen. She immediately said that would be no problem. I explained how she would never blame herself for any other crime that could have been committed, so why should she be to blame for this?

I suggested that it was a good goal for her to tell her parents, to overcome her shame.

She then said, "Could you tell them?" We discussed them coming in for a session, and I would tell them first, and then she could join the session and we could talk about it together. This way, I could help her parents understand the depth of her shame and provide more information about PTSD. She agreed, and the joint session was positive. Her parents initially had a very strong reaction of anger toward this boy and her college. They needed to process their feelings and realize that their focus had to be on supporting their daughter. They were relieved to finally know what was causing their daughter such distress. They also agreed to learn more about campus rape and PTSD.

Next Steps

When September approached, Monica was ready to go back to school, and her parents supported that decision. She sees a therapist on campus to continue the work we started. She joined a rape support group, and this is helping her blame herself less and realize she's not alone. It's also helping with her sense of shame. Telling her parents and getting their support has also helped her feel stronger and not ashamed.

Monica was right: her father's immediate reaction was wanting to kill the boy, and her mother was ready to sue the school. They were able to calm down, however, and learn more about how to help their daughter get through this. As they learned more about rape on campus, they realized that this could have happened at any school. Knowing what was bothering her all this time helped them offer her more understanding and support.

DSM-5 Guidelines

Post-Traumatic Stress Disorder

The *DSM-5* identifies the diagnostic criteria necessary for a diagnosis. The assumption is that many readers will have children who meet some but not all the criteria.

Note: The following criteria apply to adults, adolescents, and children older than 6 years. For children 6 years and younger, see corresponding criteria below.

A. Exposure to actual or threatened death, serious injury, or sexual violence in one (or more) of the following ways:

  1. Directly experiencing the traumatic event(s).

  2. Witnessing, in person, the event(s) as it occurred to others.

  3. Learning that the traumatic event(s) occurred to a close family member or close friend. In cases of actual or threatened death of a family member or friend, the event(s) must have been violent or accidental.

  4. Experiencing repeated or extreme exposure to aversive details of the traumatic event(s) (e.g., first responders collecting human remains; police officers repeatedly exposed to details of child abuse).

Note: Criterion A4 does not apply to exposure through electronic media, television, movies, or pictures, unless this exposure is work related.

B. Presence of one (or more) of the following intrusion symptoms associated with the traumatic event(s), beginning after the traumatic event(s) occurred:

1. Recurrent, involuntary, and intrusive distressing memories of the traumatic event(s).

   Note: In children older than 6 years, repetitive play may occur in which themes or aspects of the traumatic event(s) are expressed.

2. Recurrent distressing dreams in which the content and/or effect of the dream are related to the traumatic event(s).

   Note: In children, there may be frightening dreams without recognizable content.

3. Dissociative reactions (e.g., flashbacks) in which the individual feels or acts as if the traumatic event(s) were recurring. (Such reactions may occur on a continuum, with the most extreme expression being a complete loss of awareness of present surroundings.)

   Note: In children, trauma-specific reenactment may occur in play.

4. Intense or prolonged psychological distress at exposure to internal or external cues that symbolize or resemble an aspect of the traumatic event(s).

5. Marked physiological reactions to internal or external cues that symbolize or resemble an aspect of the traumatic event(s).

C. Persistent avoidance of stimuli associated with the traumatic event(s), beginning after the traumatic event(s) occurred, as evidenced by one or both of the following:

1. Avoidance of or efforts to avoid distressing memories, thoughts, or feelings about or closely associated with the traumatic event(s).

2. Avoidance of or efforts to avoid external reminders (people, places, conversations, activities, objects, situations) that arouse distressing memories, thoughts, or feelings about or closely associated with the traumatic event(s).

D. Negative alterations in cognitions and mood associated with the traumatic event(s), beginning or worsening after the traumatic event(s) occurred, as evidenced by one or both of the following:

1. Inability to remember an important aspect of the traumatic event(s) (typically due to dissociative amnesia and not to other factors such as head injury, alcohol, or drugs).

2. Persistent and exaggerated negative beliefs or expectations about oneself, others, or the world (e.g., "I am bad," "No one can be trusted," "The world is completely dangerous," "My whole nervous system is permanently ruined").

3. Persistent, distorted cognitions about the cause or consequences of the traumatic event(s) that led the individual to blame himself/herself or others.

4. Persistent negative emotional state (e.g., fear, horror, anger, guilt, or shame).

5. Markedly diminished interest or participation in significant activities.

6. Feelings of detachment or estrangement from others.

7. Persistent inability to experience positive emotions (e.g., inability to experience happiness, satisfaction, or loving feelings).

E. Marked alterations in arousal and reactivity associated with the traumatic event(s), beginning or worsening after the traumatic event(s) occurred, as evidenced by one or both of the following:

1. Irritable behavior and angry outbursts (with little or no provocation) typically expressed as verbal or physical aggression toward people or objects.

2. Reckless or self-destructive behavior.

3. Hypervigilance.

4. Exaggerated startle response.

5. Problems with concentration.

6. Sleep disturbance (e.g., difficulty falling or staying asleep or restless sleep).

F. Duration of the disturbance (Criteria B, C, D, and E) is more than 1 month.

G. The disturbance causes clinically significant distress or impairment in social, occupational, or other important areas of functioning.

H. The disturbance is not attributable to the physiological effects of a substance (e.g., medication, alcohol, or another medical condition).

Specify whether:

With dissociative symptoms: The individual's symptoms meet the criteria for post-traumatic stress disorder, and in addition, in response to the stressor, the individual experiences persistent or recurrent symptoms of either of the following:

1. **Depersonalization:** Persistent or recurrent experiences of feeling detached from, and as if one were an outside observer of, one's mental process or body (e.g., feeling as though one were in a dream; feeling a sense of unreality of self or body or of time moving slowly).

2. **Derealization:** Persistent or recurrent experiences of unreality of surroundings (e.g., the world around the individual is experienced as unreal, dreamlike, distant, or distorted).

    Note: To use this subtype, the dissociative symptoms must not be attributable to the physiological effects of a substance (e.g., blackouts, behavior during alcohol intoxication) or another medical condition (e.g., complex partial seizures).

Specify if:

With delayed expression: If the full diagnostic criteria are not met until at least 6 months after the event (although the onset and expression of some symptoms may be immediate).

Post-Traumatic Stress Disorder for Children 6 Years and Younger

A. In children 6 years and younger, exposure to actual or threatened death, serious injury, or sexual violence in one (or more) of the following ways:

1. Directly experiencing the traumatic event(s).

2. Witnessing, in person, the event(s) as it occurred to others, especially primary caregivers.

    Note: Witnessing does not include events that are witnessed only in electronic media, television, movies, or pictures.

3. Learning that the traumatic event(s) occurred to a parent or caregiving figure.

B. Presence of one (or more) of the following intrusion symptoms associated with the traumatic event(s), beginning after the traumatic event(s) occurred:

1. Recurrent, involuntary, and intrusive distressing memories of the traumatic event(s).

   Note: Spontaneous and intrusive memories may not necessarily appear distressing and may be expressed as play reenactment.

2. Recurrent distressing dreams in which the content and/or effect of the dream are related to the traumatic event(s).

3. Dissociative reactions (e.g., flashbacks) in which the child feels or acts as if the traumatic event(s) were recurring (such reactions may occur on a continuum, with the most extreme expression being a complete loss of awareness of present surroundings). Such trauma-specific reenactment may occur in play.

4. Intense or prolonged psychological distress at exposure to internal or external cues that symbolize or resemble an aspect of the traumatic event(s).

5. Marked physiological reactions to internal or external cues that symbolize or resemble an aspect of the traumatic event(s).

C. One (or more) of the following symptoms, representing either persistent avoidance of stimuli associated with the traumatic event(s) or negative alterations in cognitions and mood associated with the traumatic event(s), must be present, beginning after the event(s) or worsening after the event(s):

Persistent Avoidance of Stimuli

1. Avoidance of or efforts to avoid activities, places, or physical reminders that arouse recollections of the traumatic event(s).

2. Avoidance of or efforts to avoid people, conversations, or interpersonal situations that arouse recollections of the traumatic event(s).

Negative Alterations in Cognitions

3. Substantially increased frequency of negative emotional states (e.g., fear, guilt, sadness, shame, confusion).

4. Markedly diminished interest or participation in significant activities, including constriction of play.

5. Socially withdrawn behavior.

6. Persistent reduction in expression of positive emotions.

D. Alterations in arousal and reactivity associated with the traumatic event(s), beginning or worsening after the traumatic event(s) occurred, as evidenced by one or more of the following:

1. Irritable behavior and angry outbursts (with little or no provocation) typically expressed as verbal or physical aggression toward people or objects (including extreme temper tantrums).

2. Hypervigilance.

3. Exaggerated startle response.

4. Problems with concentration.

5. Sleep disturbance (e.g., difficulty falling or staying asleep or restless sleep).

E. Duration of the disturbance is more than 1 month.

F. The disturbance causes clinically significant distress or impairment in relationships with parents, siblings, peers, or other caregivers or with school behavior.

G. The disturbance is not attributable to the physiological effects of a substance (e.g., medication, alcohol, or another medical condition).

Specify whether:

With dissociative symptoms: The individual's symptoms meet the criteria for posttraumatic stress disorder, and the individual experiences persistent or recurrent symptoms of either of the following:

1. **Depersonalization:** Persistent or recurrent experiences of feeling detached from, and as if one were an outside observer of, one's mental process or body (e.g., feeling as though one were in a dream; feeling a sense of unreality of self or body or of time moving slowly).

2. **Derealization:** Persistent or recurrent experiences of unreality of surroundings (e.g., the world around the individual is experienced as unreal, dreamlike, distant, or distorted).

Note: To use this subtype, the dissociative symptoms must not be attributable to the physiological effects of a substance (e.g., blackouts, behavior during alcohol intoxication) or another medical condition (e.g., complex partial seizures).

With delayed expression: If the full diagnostic criteria are not met until at least 6 months after the event (although the onset and expression of some symptoms may be immediate).

American Psychiatric Association. "Posttraumatic Stress Disorder." In *Diagnostic and Statistical Manual of Mental Disorders.* 5th ed. Washington, DC: American Psychiatric Association, 2013.

Chapter 9

And There's More

Hair Pulling, Skin Picking, Tics, Picky Eating, and the Like

Disorders or habits like hair pulling and skin picking are often associated with anxiety and are frustrating for kids and parents. Helping children with these problems involves *habit reversal*, not exposure treatment, so our seven steps don't fit the way they do for the other disorders. Though the strategies differ somewhat, the treatment is still cognitive behavioral, which helps kids change the way they think and behave so that they can gain control.

Hair Pulling

Parents are often horrified and confused when they first notice their child pulling out her hair. Seeing their beautiful child with no eyelashes or eyebrows, or with bald spots on her head, can be shocking. Parents naturally respond with panic and concern about what could be causing such self-destructive behavior. It seems like there must be something terribly wrong if a child is pulling out her hair.

Parents have questions and admonitions: "Why are you doing this to yourself?" "You need to stop pulling." "Just stop doing this!"

Unfortunately, there are no easy answers. Kids don't know why they pull; they just do it. They don't want to pull and usually want desperately to stop pulling, but they can't. They feel ashamed and upset about being so out of control. They don't understand why they do it and often feel judged and misunderstood by others, especially their parents.

Kids who pull usually don't want to talk about it and even deny doing it. But parents seeing hair loss want to do something about it. The more parents want to stop the pulling, the more kids feel criticized and ashamed. This leads everyone to feel helpless and worried about the effect of the hair pulling.

Trichotillomania (trich) is the name of the condition where people pull out their hair. Most commonly, kids with this condition pull out their eyelashes, eyebrows, or head hair. Less commonly, they may pull other body hair, including pubic hair, leg hair, or arm hair.

Having a child who pulls hair is often a painful experience for parents. Mothers, in particular, are often deeply disturbed by this behavior. Hair and appearance often have more meaning and importance for women than for men, and mothers are often worried about their child being teased or bullied because of the hair loss.

Both girls and boys can have trich. It may be more common among girls, or it may be that more girls than boys seek help with it.

Parents often feel embarrassed and judged as hair loss becomes more noticeable. Among psychiatric disorders, this one usually involves the most mentally healthy kids, yet it is also the most visible to others. Parents often feel others are judging them. "What are you doing to make your child pull her hair?" Parents often blame themselves and try to figure out what they are doing wrong.

Zoey and Gary's Story

Zoey and Gary came seeking help with their 15-year-old daughter, Olivia.

"Olivia is a beautiful girl," Zoey said. "An excellent student. She gets great grades. She's an athlete—she plays hockey. She's never had any problems. About a year ago, I started noticing she looked different. Her eyebrows looked like they were getting smaller and smaller, until one morning, I looked at her, and they were totally gone. I mean gone. She had no eyebrows at all. I probably didn't react the right way. I yelled at her and said something like 'What have you done to yourself? What were you thinking to pull all your eyebrows out? Don't you ever do that again. It looks awful.'

"It was not my best parenting moment, but I was so shocked and upset. I had never seen anything like this before. Of course, Olivia burst into tears and ran out of the room. I felt terrible and tried to calm down. I told her

I was sorry for getting so upset, but I needed to know why she did this to herself. At first, she denied even doing it, then said it was an accident, then finally, after lots of tears and hugs, she admitted that she couldn't stop pulling, and she doesn't know why. Well, that really confused me. I admit, I really don't get this. It's so hard for me. I keep thinking, why would my beautiful daughter want to do this to herself?"

She composed herself and continued. "So, I knew we needed help and got her into a therapist right away. I called my insurance company, and they gave me names of therapists. I was desperate and called over fifteen. Most never got back to me. Some said they had a long waiting list. I finally got someone who took my insurance and had an appointment after school. So we met. She was very nice but admitted she didn't have much experience with this. I just wanted help for Olivia, and the therapist said she thought she could help her, and they started meeting weekly. Soon she wanted her on Prozac. I didn't want to put my child on drugs, but the therapist said it would help, so I agreed.

"Yet Olivia still had no eyebrows, and I was willing to do anything to help her. She took the Prozac, and she seemed more easygoing and relaxed. Her grades improved. She seemed happier. But still no eyebrows. When I asked her about the therapy, she said they just talked about things."

Gary then interrupted. "The reason we're here is she is now pulling her eyelashes. Maybe there's something bothering her so much she feels she needs to pull her hair out? What are we missing? This problem is getting worse even though we are doing everything we think we should do. Her therapist has no answers for us. She is very nice, but our daughter is still on medicine and now pulling not only her eyebrows but her eyelashes. This is not working. Last week, Olivia was crying. She thinks she will never have eyebrows or eyelashes. Is this true? Will they ever grow back?"

Gary didn't wait for a response. "It's bad enough she has no eyebrows, but the poor kid puts this dark powdery makeup on where her eyebrows should be. It looks awful. Sometimes I think she would look better with no eyebrows than with that fake black stuff. She's still beautiful and such a wonderful kid. I wish this didn't have to be such a big deal."

"You don't understand," Zoey cut in. "She likes boys. She wants to go to the prom. But there are school pictures, and I wonder what kids are saying about her. She may be getting teased, for all we know. That makeup does make her look very odd, but I think she would be worse if she had nothing there. Now she's pulling out her eyelashes. Eye makeup doesn't work if there are no eyelashes. Mascara can't work if there's nothing there."

Zoey looked defeated. "All this therapy and medicine, and she's worse. We don't know how to get her to stop pulling. I feel like we've tried everything and still no eyebrows."

Gary became more reflective. "It's hurting my relationship with my daughter. If I see a little improvement, I get excited, and then when it's all wiped out, I can't help it, I get so disappointed and angry. I try not to show it, but I just don't get it. Why can't she just stop pulling out her hair? We fight about it a lot, and she now just refuses to talk about it. I want to help her. I worry so much about this, but I don't know how to help her."

It was clear that we had to hear from Olivia.

Olivia's Story

I chatted with Olivia one-on-one a bit, and then she started to open up: "I began pulling my eyebrows about a year and a half ago. At first it was just a little here and there. Then one night I pulled a lot out. I didn't realize how much until I looked in the mirror. Oh my god, I was shocked. There were big gaps in my eyebrows. I felt so mad at myself. How could I have done this? And I felt embarrassed, afraid everyone was going to see what I'd done. I tried to cover it up with a little makeup, but it still showed the gaps. I prayed no one would notice, but as soon as I saw my mother, she freaked. She started yelling at me as if I did this on purpose."

She seemed distraught. "Who would want to do this? I hate it! I want to stop, but I can't. Since then, it seems the more I pull, the more I want to pull. I get urges to pull. Sometimes I look in the mirror and feel I just have to pull the hair out. Other times I could be studying or on the computer or watching TV, relaxing, and my hands go up there, and I pull without even really thinking about it. Then the damage is done, and I feel awful."

I encouraged her to continue.

"I think my mom calmed down about it a bit after she read about trichotillomania. It's such a weird name. I think she knows I don't want to do this, but I don't think she really gets it. She's always staring at my face and looking at my eyebrows. I feel we can't even have a conversation without her asking me about it or just staring. I know what she's looking at, to see if I've been pulling or if anything is growing back. It feels like that's all she thinks about now. And she always wants to talk about it. I hate that. Sometimes I wasn't even thinking about it, and she has to bring it up, and then I start thinking about it. I told her to stop it, but she can't. I know I get angry at her, and I'm not really angry at my mom. I'm angry about this whole thing. I'm angry that I pull."

"I found this powder online," she continued. "It's dark but it goes on and stays on, sort of like eyebrows. I know it doesn't look natural, but it's the best I could find. It's such an ordeal. I have to get up an hour earlier for school. I have to put it on, and sometimes it takes a long time to get it right. Then I worry all the time. I think kids are staring at my eyebrows. I try to look away from people so they won't see my face. I also worry constantly that it will get smeared, and I sometimes have to go to the bathroom at school to check that it's okay. And at hockey, I have to be so careful with the helmet not to mess up my eyebrows. I think about all this constantly. I used to be outgoing and popular. Now I feel just shy. I don't want anyone to notice me and my eyebrows. I'm constantly thinking kids are saying things about it."

She sighed deeply. "I don't know how it happened, but one night I had a lot of homework, and I had no more eyebrows to pull, so I started pulling my eyelashes. The next morning when I looked in the mirror, I was horrified. Most of my lashes were gone. I knew my mother was going to be so upset. I tried to avoid her, but she noticed. The look on her face . . . Sometimes I think she thinks I must be really crazy to be doing this. I know she was trying. She didn't yell at me, but she looked shocked, and she had tears in her eyes. She asked me about it, and I acted like I didn't know what she was talking about and quickly left for school. I hate when she asks me about this.

"I try so hard not to pull. I use squeeze balls and fidget toys, and I keep a journal about my feelings. I don't know why I do it. I hate myself after I pull. I feel like such a freak."

She said she had been to another therapist. "She kept asking what my week was like and what was making me upset. So awkward. She was nice, but I'm concerned about my hair pulling and nothing else. I started to think it was all hopeless.

"I'm afraid they won't ever grow back, and this is the way I'll always be. That really scares me. Everyone thinks it should be easy to just stop. Nobody understands how hard this is; even I don't understand why it's so hard. And I hate taking medication. It doesn't work, and if anything, the pulling is worse."

It was time to start looking for solutions, and we agreed to meet together, Olivia and her parents. Zoey, Gary, and Olivia were clearly feeling pretty hopeless. Olivia's eyebrows looked fake. Though I could tell much effort went into making them look right, under the makeup, I could tell there really weren't many hairs. Most of her eyelashes were also gone.

So we started by discussing the disorder. I explained that there is not much research on trich, due to a lack of funding and interest. Even though trich causes so much distress, it is often not viewed as a critical psychiatric problem compared to others. Add to that the shame associated with it, and finding subjects to study can be difficult. Those who are studied may not be representative of all the people who have trich.

Still, I have learned a lot about this disorder from clinical experience treating hundreds of hair pullers, and the kids I have seen who pull their hair have had several characteristics in common:

- They don't want to pull their hair. They want to stop.
- Unlike other disorders I treat, trich is not caused by anxiety. Although anxiety can be a trigger, so can boredom or being highly focused on something.
- Kids who pull often have family members who either pull their hair or pick at their skin, which lends support for a genetic component.
- Trich often comes with an obsession with hair, a hyperfocus on how hair feels and looks. Often, these kids are fidgety, their hands eager to touch and fiddle with something. For people with trich, in some ways it feels good to pull hair, since it's self-soothing. But it can quickly become a compulsive habit that feels out of control.
- Trich is not a symptom of an underlying serious psychiatric problem, but it can cause anxiety, depression, and low self-esteem. It is a burden for kids, and it carries social consequences because everybody can see it, yet it can be hard to understand.

- Kids often feel a great deal of shame about pulling and will often deny it to parents and others. Kids who never lie about anything will lie about pulling.
- It's not surprising that pulling can have a negative effect on parent-child relationships. Parents, often mothers, can feel upset about the pulling and may be desperate to stop it. They're aware of the negative social consequences pulling can have on their child. They see their child so out of control with this behavior that they want to take control and stop the pulling. Unfortunately, they can't.
- Willpower alone is usually not enough to stop the pulling, because it can be such a strong compulsive habit.
- It is very important to assess if the child is eating the hair. Although rare, some children have trichotillomania along with pica, meaning they eat the hair they pull out. These children often find hair in other places in addition to their head. For example, children with pica may eat other people's hair, pet hair, or hairs found on a brush. They are obsessed with hair and feel great satisfaction eating it. This can be very dangerous because the hair can form a ball in the stomach, called a bezoar, or a mass that would have to be removed surgically.
- Sometimes kids pull other people's hair or their pet's hair. They love their pets but can't resist pulling the hair.

The good news is, the longer a child goes without any hair pulling, the weaker the urge to pull becomes until the habit is reversed. The brain becomes retrained against pulling, and in my experience, it is extremely rare for the hair not to grow back. So even though stopping the pulling can be difficult initially, it does get easier over time.

I explained that Zoey and Gary had to stop thinking something they were doing wrong had caused this, and Olivia also had to stop blaming herself. Together they needed to work on helping Olivia stop pulling. In my experience, the most effective way to stop pulling is to make it so the child can't easily pull. This is difficult since the urge to pull is so strong. Imagine going on a diet and sitting in front of chocolate cake with a fork in your hand, or imagine trying to quit smoking with a cigarette hanging out of your mouth and a lighter in your hand. That's how hard it is to stop pulling when you have trichotillomania. Hair is always there, waiting to be pulled.

Using barriers, so the child can't feel the hair and get the grip needed to pull it, is a powerful strategy. Kids usually feel the hair before pulling it. So preventing this touching and making it hard to grip the hair to pull it can help prevent the pulling. This often entails wearing something on the fingers that takes away the ability to pull, usually Band-Aids or tape, and often gloves at night. Wearing hats, headbands, or other barriers can also be useful.

To implement this, the first step is to identify when the pulling occurs. Does the child pull throughout the day and at night, or only at certain times? Where does pulling happen? At home? In school? In bed? When on electronics? When anxious? When bored? In the car? Doing homework? In the bathroom? In front of the mirror? With tweezers? This information becomes helpful in deciding which strategies to use and when.

Olivia knew that she pulled at school, in boring classes. She also pulled in front of the TV, doing homework, when she was on her phone or the computer, and basically during her down time. Recently she had pulled some of her eyelashes in front of a mirror. Sometimes she pulled in the car, especially on long drives. She also pulled when reading. Obviously, she never pulled when playing hockey.

Kids usually pull when they are alone or feel alone. So not spending time alone is a strategy. If pulling is in front of a mirror, covering the mirror is another strategy. If tweezers are used, get rid of the tweezers. Then we look at which fingers are used to pull, usually the thumb and one or two other fingers. Covering those fingertips with Band-Aids so that kids can't grip the hair makes it impossible to pull. In addition, having the fingers covered increases awareness, because when the hand goes up to feel the hair, the Band-Aid is in the way. Wearing gloves at night can help kids who pull before going to sleep or if they wake up at night. Gloves are also helpful for morning pullers. Some pulling is so automatic and impulsive, it's almost like scratching an itch. The awareness is there a little bit, but the pulling is experienced as a thoughtless, impulsive action. Other pulling is very obsessive, with a hyperfocus on the hair and a feeling that certain hairs must be pulled. Most kids experience both impulsive and obsessive pulling. Remember that it's a self-soothing, relaxing behavior. Think of it like thumb sucking, which babies do when they're relaxed as well as when they're anxious.

As with other disorders, Olivia had to learn to "talk back" to her urge to pull. Saying no and using willpower, in addition to the strategies discussed so far, are important. She didn't automatically know what fingers she used to pull, so she put her fingers up to her eyebrows as if she were going to pull. She used two fingers on both hands. Those are the fingers that needed to be covered.

She then agreed to wear Band-Aids on her four fingers, covering the tips so that she couldn't feel the hair and couldn't pull the hair. She agreed to wear Band-Aids during the day and gloves at night. She would keep extra Band-Aids with her at school in case they fell off.

Avoiding isolation was a huge step. Her parents had never seen her pull because she always did it when she was alone or felt alone. Like most teenagers, she spent a lot of time in her room doing schoolwork and on her computer. This had to change, at least temporarily, to help her avoid pulling out her hair. So Olivia agreed to do her homework in the kitchen and not in her room for now and to try to stay out of her room as much as possible. In addition, we decided to cover the mirror in her room so it wouldn't tempt her.

Zoey and Gary agreed to remind her to wear the Band-Aids but not be the "Band-Aid Police." Olivia had to do the work herself. Nagging her about the Band-Aids will only cause friction among them. On the other hand, she was a busy girl, and she might forget, so reminding her and having lots of Band-Aids around the house could be very supportive.

I cautioned all three of them that if these strategies were used only some of the time, they would not work. There would be no progress. The behavior has to stop totally to reverse the habit, because every time Olivia pulled, she stirred up the urges all over again. Simply put, the more she pulled, the more she wanted to pull; the less she pulled, the less she wanted to pull. So to change this behavior, the practice had to completely stop.

Easier said than done. For instance, keeping fingers covered all the time can be very annoying. But it works to extinguish the behavior gradually. Over a few months, the hair usually grows back, and the desire to pull lessens. Gradually, the strategies can be decreased as the results are apparent, which increases motivation.

Incentives can also help motivate. Olivia was interested in earning money, so we discussed a system where she could earn something for every day she used these strategies. Consecutive days of implementing the strategies would get her the most money. Not pulling for an extended period would reverse this habit. Tying the incentive to the use of the Band-Aids and gloves was much better than tying it to the pulling. Kids who never lie about anything else will sometimes deny pulling because of the shame they feel. Some will say they didn't know when it happened and lie about how it happened. Arguments then can start with parents saying, "I know you pulled!" and the child saying, "I didn't pull!" Parents should not get sucked into a struggle about this; it's an argument that can't be won. Denial is a symptom of the shame. Focus on supporting the use of the strategies and measuring them, and the results should follow.

Olivia worked hard using the strategies, and she did very well. Her eyebrows and eyelashes grew back. She and her parents talked to her psychiatrist, and they all agreed to taper her off Prozac. Olivia thought it was making her tired, and no one thought it was helping with the pulling. We discussed the fact that she might become more anxious after stopping the Prozac, because it might have been alleviating her anxiety without her realizing it. Sometimes kids come off medication and then realize it was helping; other times they feel no different and are glad not to take a pill every day. Olivia was firm. She wanted to stop taking the medication.

When she stopped pulling, she became acutely aware of the burden she had endured. It had affected her socially, creating more anxiety and isolation. It had also hurt her self-esteem.

She freely expressed her relief: "I thought I was the only one who did this freaky thing. I felt like no one could understand this. I didn't understand it. I can't believe how great it feels not to have to worry about the makeup and about people looking at me all the time."

Olivia spent a lot of time every morning making sure her makeup covered the hair loss, and this had caused her to feel depressed. "It was hard not to feel hopeless about this. I kept trying to stop pulling but couldn't."

As mentioned, this behavior had certainly affected her relationship with her family, especially with her mother. "I always felt like she was looking at my eyebrows and eyelashes and judging me. Always."

Yet Olivia turned things around and did very well for many months.

Finally, she was able to suspend the strategies. After a year, however, she had a relapse and starting pulling again, which was very discouraging. Why had she slipped? She doesn't know, saying it "just happened," and she felt all the urges come back again. Fortunately, she went back to using the Band-Aids, and the pulling stopped again.

Some kids never slip; others have relapses and need to reactivate the strategies.

Olivia talked about her frustration with this. "In some ways, my mom still doesn't get it; she still thinks I do this on purpose, like I want to pull my hair. She doesn't understand how it feels. I told her, 'You know when you've had a long day, and you're exhausted, and you just feel so good putting your head down on your pillow at night? That's how it feels for me when I am pulling.'"

Children with trichotillomania, like Olivia, often say, "No one understands how hard this is." And this is why communication and education are so important.

Skin Picking

Skin picking (excoriation) is a disorder that is a lot like hair pulling, and some children do both. But with skin picking, the obsession is noticing any little imperfection, bump, or scab on the skin and feeling the need to pick at it. Kids who look like they have terrible acne may actually have minor acne, but because they feel the need to keep picking at it, it looks far worse and doesn't heal. Similarly, kids with mosquito bites may pick at the bites so much that they don't have a chance to heal.

Children with skin picking disorder can pick at their fingers, scalp, ears, face, legs, arms, feet—any place on their skin. And of course, there are kids who compulsively pick at their nose, as if their nose has to be perfectly clean inside.

A major problem with skin picking is the risk of infection. In these days of super bugs that are resistant to antibiotics, infections are not something to take lightly. When a child picks, putting antibiotic cream on the area and seeking medical attention if there's even a question of it being infected is important.

Like hair pulling, skin picking often runs in the family, and the strategies used are similar: barriers to make it difficult to pick, such as long-sleeve shirts and pants, Band-Aids on the picking fingers and sometimes on the area picked; keeping the skin clean; and having things to fidget with to prevent picking.

Among the scores of children I have treated for skin picking is the experience of Liam.

Nevan and Pete's Story

Nevan and Pete saw me about their 7-year-old son. "Liam has always been a nail biter and picked at his fingers, but lately it's gotten worse," Nevan told me. "He's been picking his nose, which I know is such a terrible habit. In the last couple of months, he started having nose bleeds, which he never had before. So we took him to the pediatrician. He admitted to the doctor that he's been picking his nose, and this is causing the nose bleeds.

"We realized then, this is serious. Nothing we say or do seems to make a difference. We tell him to stop, that he's going to get teased, that it's dirty, that he can get an infection if he keeps picking. Sometimes I don't even think he's aware he's doing it. If we punish him, it doesn't work. It's like he can't stop himself. We found bloody tissues in the bathroom the other night, and I'm sure it was from his picking."

Pete added, "He also picks at his feet at night, and if he gets a mosquito bite, forget it. He can't seem to leave it alone. When he was younger, he used to chew his clothes, but that's stopped. I've caught him picking at his head; at one point hair was missing, because he was picking so much. And one more spot, I know this is weird, but right inside his ear, he picks at sometimes, and that can lead to a scab. I know it's just a matter of time before kids start to make fun of him or he gets an infection. We don't know how to get him to stop."

I explained that we could implement strategies, and we decided to all meet together.

Liam's Story

Liam was a little fidgety in his chair as we started, but he was honest. "I know I pick. I can't help it. I feel like when I have a scab, I just have to pick it until it's gone. Any bump I feel, I need to pick at it. Lately it's been my nose. I feel like there's something in there, and I have to pick and pick until I get everything out. Then a couple of weeks ago, all this blood came out, and it scared me. I thought something was really wrong. Now it's happened a few times. I can't stop picking, and I know it's gross, but I feel like I have to do it. Sometimes I don't even realize I'm doing it, and my mom and dad will yell at me to stop. They get angry at me and sometimes grab my hand to get me to stop. I try to stop when they tell me to, but then it starts up again. It feels like they're always nagging at me to stop. In school, sometimes I feel like I just have to pick my nose, so I do it so nobody sees me. I sneak it so the kids don't see me do it."

As with hair pulling, we needed to initiate strategies to help Liam stop picking. Since the dynamics of picking and pulling are very similar, so are the strategies to reverse the habits. A Band-Aid on the picking finger forms a barrier and is particularly effective for nose picking. Plus it increases awareness, which is important because kids who pick often don't realize they're doing it.

Other strategies include a Band-Aid on skin that was picked at, long-sleeve shirts and pants if the picking is on the arms and legs, and a tight-fitting shirt if the picking is on the back or chest. Some kids pick their feet, but this is usually at night, and socks can be a barrier. Many kids pick their head, and a hat or a headband that covers the picking spot serves as a barrier.

Naturally, children who pick have to resist the urge so that the urges gradually lessen. They particularly need to understand that taking care of the open wounds from picking is crucial because infections can be dangerous.

Liam agreed to wear a Band-Aid on his picking fingers, wear socks at night, and try hard to stop his picking. He agreed to wear a baseball cap to help with his head picking. He also agreed to let his parents be aware of any spots he's been picking at, so they can monitor for infections.

For incentives, we discussed earning points every day for using the strategies, with big bonus points for successful consecutive days. As the points accumulated, Liam got closer to the prize of going to a baseball game with his dad.

I emphasized that not picking for many days in a row was what would reverse the habit.

Liam, like Olivia, worked really hard to reverse the habit and did a good job, with less and less picking. After a couple of months, he didn't need the strategies anymore. But if he slips, he knows he has to go back to wearing the Band-Aids until the urge passes.

Like most conditions, skin picking and hair pulling can be mild, moderate, or severe, and more strategies and closer monitoring are needed when the problem is severe.

Tics

Tics are involuntary movements or vocalizations that are associated with Tourette syndrome and transient tic disorder. Some kids have what look like classic tics, but the tics are more anxiety-driven, obsessive compulsive movements. Many kids have both: tics that are involuntary or thoughtless as well as other movements they feel they "have to do." These latter tics are more obsessive and in a sense voluntary. Understanding which kind of tics a child experiences is important because both the CBT technique and the appropriate medications are different for tics than for OCD.

Anxiety-driven, obsessive movements often look like classic tics. These can include eye rolling, head shaking, mouth movements, breathing rituals, sniffing, and vocalizations. How do you tell the difference? I have learned to ask the children and listen to the parents. Parents often have a sense of how much control their children have over these movements. And asking the children what makes them do these things often provides a clue to how voluntary the movements are.

True tics are like hiccups: they just happen without the person thinking about it. More obsessive movements happen for a reason, although the reason is irrational. The CBT treatment for tics is called habit reversal training and does not involve exposure response prevention (ERP), which is most effective with anxiety-driven movements. (See chapter 6 for a description of ERP.)

Kids with tics are often very accepting of them. It can be more difficult for parents who are watching their child's tics. For parents, often the best approach is to accept the tics, knowing that the child will most likely outgrow them.

Sometimes tics are severe and can cause the child distress or discomfort. Fortunately, habit reversal training has been found to be an effective treatment. This training involves increasing awareness and developing a "competing movement" that the child can apply to fight tics. Practicing this technique generally helps reduce tics; medication can sometimes help as well.

Sally, 7 years old, had generalized anxiety. She had a fear of choking that developed into a fear of not getting enough air. She would take frequent short quick breaths that seemed like tics. Her mother insisted that this habit was not a tic, that it was based on her fear: "She will be rapidly breathing periodically, which seems automatic and thoughtless. For example, when we are having a conversation, or when she is relaxed and playing. The rapid breathing started with a fear, but she has been gasping so often, it has become a habit."

We worked on Sally "talking back to the worries." Her fears were worse when she had a cold, because she then worried more about her breathing. She made progress with this approach but was also put on antianxiety medication by another doctor. This combination caused the "breathing tic" to disappear, as did her fear of not getting enough air. Her mother was right: It was an anxiety-based movement and not a tic.

A teenage boy I worked with had head-shaking and hand-wiping movements and vocalizations. He had been diagnosed with Tourette syndrome. He was taking medication to help reduce his tics. As I met with him, however, it became clear that these were obsessive compulsive movements that looked like tics. He explained, "When I get a 'bad' thought, I have to cancel it out by shaking my head. When I see kids I don't like—you know, the kids who do drugs and don't do well in school—when I walk by them or even think of their names, I have to shake my body. I know it sounds weird, but it feels like if I don't do this, I could turn into them, or be like them, so I have to shake, sometimes just my head, sometimes my whole body. Then if I touch something they have touched, I have to wipe my hands on something, you know, wipe it off."

He also mumbled under his breath sometimes. When asked about that, he said, "When I get a bad thought I have to say my name quickly three times to cancel out the thoughts."

His treatment consisted of exposure response prevention because these "tics" were really OCD rituals. He stopped his tic medication because he didn't have Tourette syndrome.

I worked with this young man to help him not do the movements while looking at the kids who triggered him to do the movements. Then we worked on him intentionally having a "bad thought" (which for him was either sexual or violent) and not doing the vocalizations. The exposure to the kids and to the thoughts took the power out of them and made it easier for him to stop doing his movements. One by one, he was able to stop all his movements and vocalizations.

As noted above, sometimes treatment can be complicated because kids can have both tics and anxiety-driven movements. A boy I worked with had eye tics, including blinking and eye rolling. When asked about it, he explained that the blinking just happens. "I don't even know I'm doing it. But the other thing, with my eyes, that's different. If I see something in the corner of my eye, I feel I have to roll my eye back and forth. It's kinda like needing to even it out."

One eye movement, the blinking, is a tic; the other is an obsessive compulsive movement. I never would have known that if I hadn't asked him about it, because they both looked like classic eye tics. The treatment for the eye rolling was exposure response prevention. He worked on intentionally seeing something in the corner of his eye and not doing the eye rolling. He was able to work on that successfully, and the movement went away.

He still has the eye-blinking tic, but that doesn't bother him.

Picky Eating

Many kids restrict what foods they will eat, but when this behavior is extreme, it may be anxiety based. When children have no physical reasons for eating difficulties, yet they limit their food choices dramatically, anxiety is likely at the root of the problem. If we think of anxious kids as wanting to stay in their comfort zone and not wanting to try new things, or take risks, it makes sense that this can be applied to food. Parents often become alarmed because the food selections can be so limited.

An example of this is 8-year-old Jackson, who has generalized anxiety. His diet consists primarily of pasta with butter, but it has to be Ronni pasta shells. He will eat pizza, from one pizza restaurant, with no cheese. Jackson also eats chicken nuggets and fries, but only from McDonald's. In addition, he eats raw carrot sticks and grapes. He used to eat cheese, but not anymore. Recently, he has started eating sugar puff cereal. That's his entire diet, and he refuses to try any other foods except, like most kids with this problem, sweets—he will gladly eat candy, cookies, and cake.

What helped Jackson expand his palate was graduated exposure with incentives. This included eating some nonpreferred food before he was able to eat his preferred food. He was involved in the choices of food, but he had to eat the nonpreferred food repeatedly until he became more used to it and was able to incorporate it into his diet.

Of course, parents can play a large role in this problem. Some parents are extremely tolerant of picky eating and may make different meals for each child. Other parents are more concerned and able to be more firm in their approach to eating. With an anxious child, the sooner we work on this, the better. Eating a variety of healthy foods is learned behavior that starts very early in life. Avoidance of new foods, just like avoidance of new experiences, should not be permitted in an anxious child.

Stomach Problems, Constipation, and Headaches

Another anxiety-related behavior is the problem of constipation, a common problem with anxious children. Young children can be afraid of having a bowel movement and may withhold it until they are "backed up." Often they need to take a stool softener daily, to make it easier for them. Once they are constipated, it can become a vicious cycle, because having a bowel movement then becomes painful, causes avoidance, and results in further constipation.

Using a stool softener and having sitting times on the toilet is the best approach. Of course, parents have to monitor bowel movements so that constipation doesn't develop into a chronic problem. I also encourage them to work closely with their pediatrician.

We all know that tension can cause headaches, and among anxious children, headaches can be a real concern. Relaxing, staying hydrated, and eating a balanced diet can help keep headaches under control. As with all anxiety-related physical problems, reducing the anxiety lessens the problem. When needed, pain medication can also be used. It's important to keep the headaches from interfering with a child's functioning. Kids have to learn to ignore the pain and keep active.

The same with stomach pains. Kids have to recognize that these pains are "the worries" and not a sign that they are sick. They need to push themselves to continue their activities; often the distraction helps the pain go away. In addition, by "pushing through their anxiety," kids find out that the anxiety decreases, and with that, the pain decreases. Physical problems caused by anxiety should not be used as a reason to avoid anxiety-producing situations.

More Reasons for Hope

Although the above conditions aren't classic anxiety disorders and don't easily lend themselves to the seven steps, they can be extremely frustrating. The good news is that cognitive behavioral techniques can solve these issues and help children and their parents move on.

Chapter 10

....

Easier Said Than Done

When More Help Is Needed

Anxiety disorders can be mild, moderate, or severe. When applying cognitive behavioral therapy (CBT) strategies at home is not enough, professional guidance is often needed. But be forewarned: the mental health system for children can feel like a maze that is difficult to navigate. There are social workers, mental health counselors, school counselors, psychologists, nurse practitioners, and psychiatrists. If that's not confusing enough, there are different kinds of therapies, from play therapy to talk therapy, family therapy to biofeedback, psychoanalytical therapy to mindfulness therapy, cognitive behavioral therapy (CBT) to dialectical behavior therapy (DBT).

My considered preference is CBT because it is evidence based, meaning that much research has been done proving its effectiveness, especially for children with anxiety disorders.

Psychiatrists are medical doctors who have a medical degree (MD) and specialize in treating psychological disorders with medication. Some child psychiatrists provide medication and therapy; some focus only on prescribing the right medication for children. Child psychiatrists are very skilled in understanding psychiatric medications and choosing among many different choices for individual children and adolescents. Most therapists have relationships with psychiatrists they trust. Therapists can guide you if they feel medication should be added to your child's treatment, though medications should be the last treatment option in most cases, not the first. If your child is severely ill or at risk of serious harm to self or others, including talking about doing harm, you should seek immediate medical care for your child.

Finding a Therapist

Unfortunately, there are many therapists who say they do CBT with kids after they have taken a weekend workshop in it, and the truth is that their training is limited. Therefore, you need to meet with any potential therapist for your child and feel comfortable with that person. I recommend meeting first without your child, so you can more freely discuss your child's problems and ask questions about the therapist's approach.

For instance:

- What is your training?
- Are you licensed?
- How much experience do you have doing CBT with children?
- How much do you involve the parents in this process?
- How will we be able to judge if it is working?
- What is the cost, and do you take my insurance?
- How often will you meet with my child?
- Do you have after-school and/or weekend hours?
- Now that you know some of my child's difficulties, what is your approach?

Social workers and mental health therapists usually have one to two years of schooling after their BA or BS. Psychologists have at least four years of graduate schooling, plus an internship, dissertation, and postdoctoral study. A social worker with extensive clinical experience and training in CBT, however, could be a better fit for a particular child or problem than a psychologist who specialized in research and has far less clinical training. As in any field, there are good people who know what they're doing, and there are other good people, with less training and experience, who are not as competent. You want someone who is skilled and experienced in CBT and who will involve you in understanding how the process works.

You also want to be able to see measurable progress. Although there are plenty of well-meaning professionals your child can chat with, you want to ensure that the right treatment is being provided to reduce your child's anxiety.

Recommendations from friends and from your child's pediatrician can be good sources for finding a therapist. You probably know people whose children have been in therapy, and these personal recommendations can be useful. Schools also can be a resource for referrals to a therapist, if you feel comfortable sharing this need with your child's guidance counselor.

When you meet with the therapist, trust your feelings. Do you feel comfortable that this is a good match? Will the therapist do an assessment and give you a diagnosis? Many parents seek therapy for their child because they want help and because they want to know what's wrong. A diagnosis is a starting point in understanding how to help your child.

Also keep in mind, once you engage with a therapist, you are not married to that person. If you don't feel it's working, or are not feeling comfortable, it's fine to find another therapist who is a better match. Never worry about a therapist's feelings when it comes to this issue. Finding the right match for your child is most important in making the therapy work.

Deciding on Medication

When a child has an infection or other physical medical problem, a responsible parent will seek and administer appropriate medication. No responsible parent will hastily medicate their child to treat anxiety, however. For most parents, it's a very difficult decision to make. I think medication should be considered, under certain circumstances, but not as a first line of treatment. When anxiety is severe, it can be too hard for children to apply the CBT strategies and do the necessary work because they are so flooded with overwhelming feelings. Severe anxiety can be crippling to a child and very painful, and for these children, medication plus therapy may be needed.

When should an evaluation for antianxiety medications be considered? Consider the following three examples:

1. When the anxiety is so severe that it's interfering with the health of the child

An example is a teenage girl I worked with who had a severe phobia of choking that caused her to stop eating. She was rapidly losing weight, and although we were making progress getting her to drink and eat bits of soft foods, it wasn't enough. It was so hard for her to challenge this fear and eat. So medication was added, and she made significant, rapid progress. The medication made it possible for her to realize how irrational her fear was. Gaining that insight helped her eat more and enabled us to continue the therapy.

Another example is a little girl with severe separation anxiety. She had been doing CBT, but her anxiety was pervasive. The anxiety started triggering headaches and exhausting her. She said, "Mommy, it's just so hard, and I'm only 11 years old." Medication made a big difference in reducing her anxiety and her headaches.

2. When the anxiety is so severe that it's interfering with the child's functioning, including the ability to respond to CBT

The "exposure" for these children with severe anxiety is simply to get through the day. They can't function because they are paralyzed by irrational anxiety. Severe anxiety may have psychotic features. Gaining insight and applying the cognitive strategies of challenging anxious thoughts may be impossible. Medication added to therapy can help the child be better able to apply the CBT.

A good illustration of this is children who have school phobia, with significant trouble attending school. These situations are often complicated and demand coordination with family and school, but medication to help the child feel less anxious can make the difference needed to get the child to school.

3. When kids are so anxious, they are often angry, with panic attacks and explosive behavior that interferes with family life

When the anxiety seems pervasive and is not responding enough to CBT, adding medication can make a big difference.

For instance, I worked with a 12-year-old who was very anxious and angry and took it out on her family, especially her mother. The medication decreased her anxiety, and because she was feeling more comfortable and less anxious, her anger lessened. Adding medication made a big difference for her and her family. Her father said, "I have my daughter back."

Are kids overmedicated? Many are, since medication can be seen as a quick fix. Insurance companies, when approving therapy sessions, often routinely ask if a medication evaluation was done, and if not, why not? Frankly, covering the cost of medication can be cheaper than covering the cost for therapy. But giving children medication for anxiety without therapy gives children the wrong message. Pills can't take the place of working to manage anxiety. This is a very important point: children are working and learning useful skills, and medication can help them apply these skills. My concern about medication without therapy is that children don't learn about themselves and how to control their feelings; rather, they put their faith in a pill instead. Not a great message to grow up with.

Medications also may come with side effects. Most kids are easy to medicate, and a low dose of a medication can make a big difference, sometimes with no side effects. Yet other kids have major side effects, so finding the right medication or combination of medications can be a challenge. Unfortunately, no one knows who will be easy, and who will be difficult, to medicate. And yes, these medications are powerful: they work on the brain. Therefore, children starting on a medication for anxiety need to be carefully monitored for side effects. When side effects occur, one medication is usually discontinued and replaced by another.

Unlike some other medications, where the choices and dosing are standard, antianxiety medications vary considerably from child to child. A small child may need a high dose of a medication to get a positive response, and a big teenager may need a low dose of the exact same medication. Two children with identical anxiety symptoms may have totally different reactions to the medications aimed at alleviating those symptoms. Prescribing these medications is more of an art than a science, so it's important to work with a doctor who is very experienced and knowledgeable about these medications.

Some pediatricians are comfortable prescribing medications for anxiety; others are not. If it appears to be a "simple" solution, and the pediatrician's initial medication works, that's great. But if it becomes more complicated, most pediatricians will refer to a child psychiatrist or nurse practitioner who specializes in medications for anxious kids. This is their expertise. They don't prescribe for infections and fevers; they prescribe only for psychiatric illnesses. They are the specialists who know these medications, in contrast to the pediatrician, who is a generalist. Overall, while a generalist may be fine in some circumstances, sometimes a specialist is needed.

The most common medications prescribed for children with anxiety disorders are selective serotonin reuptake inhibitors (SSRI). Believed to increase the level of the neurotransmitter serotonin, they are taken daily and may take several weeks before the effects are felt. Children usually start with a very low dose, and several weeks later, if no response, the dose is increased as needed. This interval continues until the dose is making a difference in reducing the anxiety. Many kids are on these medications for only nine months to a year, though some are on them longer. The younger the child, the more conservative I am about the use of medications. I also prefer to attempt to get kids off medications when they have an extended time of being symptom-free. I never assume children have to stay on medications for the rest of their lives.

A common side effect of the SSRIs can be sexual dysfunction—reduced arousal and difficulty having an orgasm—for both women and men. This information is not frequently shared with teenagers, because we like to think they don't have sex. However, it's an important side effect to discuss with them. I'm sure many kids who have been on these drugs through puberty have had a diminished sex drive but didn't realize it. Very little is known about how that diminished sex drive affects their development and feelings about themselves.

The other class of medications that is sometimes used for anxiety is benzodiazepines. They enhance the effect of the neurotransmitter gamma-aminobutyric acid (GABA), resulting in a sedative, sleep-inducing, anticonvulsant and muscle-relaxing effect. They can be short or long acting, and they do not take long to take effect, unlike the SSRIs. The anxiety-reducing effect is felt right away. Short-term use of these medications, or using them "as needed," is most common. Long-term use is not generally advised due to their addictive qualities. These drugs can be abused, unlike the SSRIs, because they have immediate antianxiety effects.

In addition, melatonin, which is a hormone sold over the counter (without a prescription) in health food stores and pharmacies, in the vitamin section, is often used to help kids sleep. If your child has difficulty falling asleep and gets more anxious before sleep, melatonin can be a useful sleep aid. It is natural and does not require a prescription. Check with your child's doctor about the appropriate dose. *Always discuss this and all medications with your child's pediatrician.*

School Involvement

When is it necessary to get help from your child's school?

It's important to involve your child's school when the anxiety shows itself at school and when school performance is affected. You want the school to understand your child, and there may be supports the school can offer. If the anxiety is only evident when your child is at home, and there are no symptoms at school, the school doesn't have to be involved.

I have worked with many anxious children who are very disruptive at home but are model students at school. Alice, an 8-year-old with OCD, is a good example of this. She couldn't wear underwear, had night rituals that sometimes brought her mother to tears, experienced anxiety-driven tantrums at home, and was so rigid in her thinking that any change in plans caused a meltdown. When her mother went to her teacher conference, the teacher said that she wished all her students were like Alice, who was a role model for others. Needless to say, her mother almost fell off her chair. Even though that was surprising to her mother, there was no need to involve the school, because she was fine there. Sometimes the structure, consistency, and predictability of school is containing for anxious children, in a way that home life can't be.

Jacob, a 6-year-old with selective mutism, is the opposite. He's fine at home, happy, a normal kid; all his anxiety is school focused. At school he's silent and withdrawn. His school has to be directly involved and give him a lot of supports to help him talk more and be less anxious.

School Bullying

Many anxious children have a lot of school-based social anxiety that can severely affect their school performance. Kids spend a great deal of time in school, interacting with their peers. These interactions are not always positive, and when toxic, they can create intense anxiety. Issues of bullying are unfortunately all too common. Bullying can take the form of a child being targeted and harassed or excluded in hurtful ways. Victims of bullying often feel helpless and overwhelmed because they have to face a hostile school environment every day. Bullies can be sneaky, with so much of their behavior happening off the teacher's radar. This dynamic can create intense anxiety for a child.

The issue of cyberbullying remains an ongoing problem among kids through the role of social media. Kids may write mean things they would never say to another child face to face. The written word is often very public, read by large groups of kids who get involved rapidly in the group chat. The intensity of this interaction is amazing because anything written is read and often responded to quickly by many kids. Within minutes, a child can feel violated by a crowd of kids and feel overwhelmed and unable to respond.

I have worked with girls, often in middle school, in situations where fifteen girls are online chatting, saying very mean things about one particular girl. Sometimes it takes the form of online battles among groups of girls, almost like schoolyard fighting, only far more intense. Unlike the spoken word, the written word lasts forever, for anyone to see. Not having face-to-face contact during these fights elevates the cruelty. Understandably, these exchanges can cause severe anxiety. Words are written and read, but the writing doesn't show the faces of sadness and fear these kids feel; it doesn't reveal the sound of the crying among these girls. Words can be very cold, and without face-to-face communication, so much is missed. These increasingly common experiences can be overwhelming for children and the cause not only of panic attacks, but of suicidal feelings.

Schools need to be actively involved in promoting a less hostile environment for kids, and parents should alert the administration when these things are happening. Kids need to be held accountable for bullying behavior, and there needs to be a zero-tolerance policy. Kids also need to be taught that whatever they write is public—that there is no privacy.

School Stress

Schools sometimes also play a role in increasing anxiety among kids. The pressure to excel, the excessive homework load, and "teaching to the test" all can contribute to overwhelming anxiety. Middle school kids start worrying about getting into the "right college." High school kids often can't possibly get the amount of sleep they need for their health because of the homework load. Many of them fall asleep at school, or wish they could. Schools and communities have to look at how the culture is causing kids to be far more anxious than they should be, and they need to work to promote a healthier environment for kids. With more progress in this area, I believe we would see fewer children not only on antianxiety medications, but also on stimulants to stay focused and alert.

504 Plans and IEPs for Anxious Children

Anxiety is a medical illness, and anxious children who need accommodations can request a 504 Plan. This is a legal document that guarantees your child certain accommodations due to a medical illness.

Many parents are also familiar with IEPs (Independent Educational Plans), which are for children who have difficulty accessing the curriculum due to learning disabilities or more severe social and emotional problems. An IEP may be appropriate if a child needs intensive support to learn, including placement in a more therapeutic school setting. A 504 Plan is more common for children who have anxiety disorders and provides accommodations to help them manage their anxiety in school.

Common accommodations that anxious kids may require include:

- Extra time for tests
- Extended deadlines for homework
- Ability to take breaks when needed
- Ability to meet regularly with the school counselor
- Frequent communication between parents and teacher concerning anxiety
- Ability to meet with the teacher before school starts in the fall
- Ability to have friends in the same class
- Ability to be excused from class participation as needed
- Reduced homework load
- Ability to eat outside the cafeteria
- Ability to use the nurse's bathroom
- Ability to have a counselor-led social group, often called "lunch bunch"

The hope is that kids will need less of the above as they work on reducing their anxiety. These supports can be crucial, however, to help children feel less anxious at school. School counselors can be a huge support when anxiety situations result at school, because they know the peers and the teachers and are right there to help. Many kids who have social anxiety or school anxiety can benefit from a counselor who is on site and able to help, in addition to an outside therapist.

When to Get a Neuropsychological Evaluation

When children appear to be struggling at school and showing a lot of anxiety, it's easy to attribute the school difficulties to the anxiety. But kids can be complicated. If there is an underlying undiagnosed learning disability or problems with attention and focus, an already anxious child becomes far more anxious. Imagine an anxious child, sitting in a classroom, and not understanding what the teacher is teaching, or an anxious child spacing out and having no idea what's going on in the classroom. These situations could trigger panic in an already anxious child.

Too often the focus of all problems is on the child's anxiety. But the anxiety could be a normal reaction to a difficult school situation. Having a comprehensive neuropsychological evaluation can tease out what's anxiety and what might be something else going on with your child. Understanding your child's needs can help guide treatment decisions and decide what supports your child may need at school. As noted earlier, your child may need supports in the form of an IEP. The neuropsychological evaluation can help determine if that's what's needed, and if so, how to get it for your child.

These evaluations should be done by a licensed neuropsychologist, trained and experienced in working with children. They should include an IQ test; achievement tests; tests of attention, organization, memory, and processing speed; psychological assessments; and other tests, depending on the questions needing answers. As a parent, you should expect to receive a comprehensive report outlining the tests conducted and the results, and providing a summary and recommendations for your child. Testing results can help you understand your child's cognitive and emotional functioning as well as how best to support your child.

Many parents seek independent neuropsychologists, who usually provide a far more comprehensive evaluation, and as a result, they may make different conclusions and recommendations. Parents have a right to bring this information to their child's school and expect their child's educational needs to be met.

Parent as Advocate: Working with Your Child's School

It can feel very frustrating to see your child suffering with anxiety, clearly needing more school support and not getting it. Parents can hire advocates who know the laws and your rights in relation to your child's school-based needs. It's not something everyone wants to do, but sometimes hiring an advocate can be a useful way to get what your child needs from the school system. In addition, attorneys may be useful in advocating for your child.

When to Get More Medical Tests

When a child with anxiety presents with headaches or stomachaches, anxiety may be the cause of these pains. It's important to involve a pediatrician, however, especially if children experience these problems when they're not anxious. I always feel more comfortable ruling out a medical cause for physical symptoms before assuming they're anxiety based.

A good example is an 11-year-old boy who had OCD and lots of anxiety. He also complained randomly of stomach pain, but his complaints didn't always come when he was anxious; in fact, he sometimes complained when he was having fun with friends. It was easy to assume it was his anxiety causing his pain, since anxiety often causes stomach discomfort. His parents pursued this with his pediatrician, and I recommended that they follow up further. And sure enough, tests revealed that this boy had celiac disease. With a change in his diet, the stomach pain disappeared.

On the other hand, I have also worked with kids whose physical pain was an expression of their anxiety and who underwent too many medical tests to find a physical cause. Tests that come back normal are a sign that anxiety is the cause of the pain. This can become a vicious cycle. Anxiety causes the pain, and the pain causes anxiety, which causes more hyperfocus on the pain and even more anxiety. There are always more tests that can be done, and knowing where to draw the line on medical tests is important.

Sometimes the expression of pain really is caused by the anxiety, or becomes a way to avoid anxious situations. Saying, "I'm sick," is for many kids easier and more effective than saying, "I'm worried and scared." And parents often respond differently, with more patience and support, to sick kids than to anxious kids. As parents, if we think our children are truly in pain, we don't want to push them. Many anxious kids know this and complain about pain to avoid anxiety-producing situations. Sorting this out as a parent is not always easy. A child who uses sickness as an avoidance strategy is a very anxious child who can look comfortable and relaxed when avoiding situations and challenges.

Parents have to become aware that their child is "faking it" out of the desperate need to avoid challenging situations, which can include social activities, extracurricular activities, and in the worst cases, attending school. Anxiety can cause children to become very "manipulative" due to the intense need to avoid feeling anxious.

Alternative Approaches

Tools that promote relaxation can be useful for children as well as adults. Physical exercise can reduce anxiety and improve mood. So having your child involved in regular aerobic exercise can be as powerful as medication for anxiety. In addition, kids today spend so much time in front of screens; they are often not getting the exercise they need. Being away from a screen and being involved in other activities is important, not just for a child's physical health, but for a child's mental health as well.

Making sure your child is getting enough sleep is also very important. With too little sleep, kids may become more anxious. So many kids are sleep deprived, especially teenagers. Without enough sleep, children are at greater risk for anxiety, mood, and attentional disorders. Kids need their sleep, and with computer games and social media often done in isolation—without parents knowing if the child is sleeping—sleep is often sacrificed.

Overuse of screens can be a huge problem for anxious kids. It allows them to avoid healthier activities. Sleep, exercise, and social activities need to take priority over the use of screens. Parents need to set limits and follow through with those limits so anxious kids can't hide for hours every day behind screens. And "virtual friends" are not the same as face-to-face, real-life friends. Kids need to be with other kids away from screens.

Depending on the child, meditation and yoga can also offer relief from anxiety symptoms. In addition, biofeedback is a structured way of teaching children how to relax their bodies; depending on the child, biofeedback can be useful.

When Parents Need Support

Parenting an anxious child can be challenging for many reasons. For one, these children can be demanding of time and energy. When the anxiety symptoms are severe or include more explosive behaviors, the whole family is affected. Since anxiety is contagious, the atmosphere in the family of an anxious child can become intense and stressed.

Parents of anxious children often feel overwhelmed and in need of support. For some parents, this experience causes them to seek therapy and even medication for themselves. They may benefit from guidance to keep their anxiety under control. Sometimes parents have conflicts with each other about how to parent their anxious child. Disagreeing about when to push and when to be more protective of the child is common. Knowing how hard to push, and how much to protect, can be confusing. When one parent is more firm and another more lenient, parents who don't fight about anything else may argue about their anxious child. When your child feels out of control, it's easy to blame each other. Many couples consider therapy to help resolve conflicts about parenting. It strengthens the ability to support each other and can be beneficial, not only to the parents, but to the whole family.

There are support groups for almost everything but few support groups for parents of anxious children. Why? There's a great stigma about any kind of mental illness, including one as common as anxiety. As mentioned before, many anxious kids are high functioning, so they often have a hard time integrating their sense of being so "normal" with having an anxiety disorder. They may not want anyone to know they have anxiety, because they feel ashamed.

Many of my teenage patients suffering with severe irrational fears are also successful students, fine athletes, and popular kids. They often say, "None of my friends would ever believe I'm sitting here in a therapist's office. Everyone thinks it's the weird kids who need this help. I'm not one of the weird kids."

I understand how these kids feel and why they want to keep it all very private. Yet another part of me hopes that more anxious kids will speak up about their struggles, because that's what will help break down the stigma. It will also demonstrate to others how many "normal" kids suffer from anxiety disorders and affirm that it's not something to feel ashamed about.

Parents are also aware of the stigma about mental illness, and often want to protect their child from any negative consequences that might follow if others know about their child's anxiety. They don't want their child to be harshly judged, and they don't want to be judged as bad parents. When a child has a mental health problem, many people still believe that the parents must be doing something wrong.

One of the parents I work with noted that parents of autistic children certainly have their own challenges, but they are not blamed the way parents of children with psychiatric problems are blamed. Autism is understood to be biologically based and not caused by bad parenting. The same acceptance isn't offered to parents of children with psychiatric problems, even though these problems are also biologically based. As a result, parents of anxious children often suffer in silence, not wanting others to blame them for their child's problems and not wanting others to know what they're going through.

The notion that all children are born the same, and some children simply end up with anxiety or other problems because of bad parenting, is incorrect. The idea that kids who are calm and relaxed are that way because of superior parenting is also incorrect. Clearly, kids are born with different wiring. The proof of this is how often, in the same family with the same parents, one child can be calm and anxiety-free, and the other can be the polar opposite. One child makes parenting look like a breeze, while the other is far more challenging and demanding.

A 10-year-old patient with anxiety and explosive behavior was disruptive in his church group. Parents complained, and he was asked to leave. His mom was naturally very upset, especially because she had a long relationship with this church, and her son liked going to the classes. Yet she understood, she said, "I used to be one of those mothers. I hate to say it, but back then, I would've complained. Before I went through this with my son, I had no clue."

The isolation that parents feel, the sense that no one really "gets it," can be profound. The stigma of so many other things in our society has been discarded, but the stigma of having a child with any kind of mental illness lives on.

This stigma can be broken only if we break it together, through educating others and sharing with friends and family what it's really like to parent an anxious child. Speak up when people give you well-meaning but annoying advice, like "Why don't you just tell her to relax?" "Ah, if only I'd thought of that." Explain that if it were that easy, there'd be no problem. People need to be educated about anxiety. The more parents talk openly about their challenges with anxiety, the more support they will find, because this is an epidemic that affects so many families.

Parents of anxious children could be a more effective resource for each other. Navigating the mental health system alone is a challenge. What if parents shared information about their helpful therapists and talked about strategies they've found effective with their children? Lending support, breaking down the myths, and feeling less alone as your family is turned upside-down by anxiety could be of great benefit. To do this, parents have to confront the stigma about having an anxious child.

What could this look like? Monthly meetings led by parents on a rotating basis, with community speakers and time allotted so parents can share stories and suggestions. This sounds easy, but when you're exhausted with an anxious child and everything else, it's not so easy. I believe that community mental health centers and schools could offer more of this kind of support, in coordination with parents. These meetings could also help the wider community examine ways to decrease children's anxiety on a broader scale.

In short, the epidemic of anxious children demands that kids learn how to manage their anxiety, that parents learn how to help them, and that communities learn what they can do to reduce anxiety among their youth. We all have to share in the responsibility for this problem affecting our kids.

Acknowledgments

I offer sincere thanks to the following individuals. Without their contributions and support, this book would not have been written.

I am grateful to Gary Woonteiler and Woonteiler Ink for editing and writing support, Dr. Jerome Rogoff for ongoing support, Margaret Sharkey for cheering me on, Lisa Tener for her amazing voice giving form to this book, Regina Brooks for believing in this project, and Jackie Wehmueller, who brought this book to press.

And my thanks also go, as always, to my patients—my greatest teachers—who have allowed me the privilege of getting to know them, laughing with them, and helping them overcome anxiety.

Notes

1. Jane E. Costello, Helen L. Egger, and Adrian Angold, "The Developmental Etiology of Anxiety Disorders: Phenomenology, Prevalence, and Comorbidity," in *Phobic and Anxiety Disorders in Children and Adolescents: A Clinician's Guide to Effective Psychosocial and Pharmacological Interventions*, ed. Thomas Ollendick and John March, 61–92 (New York: Oxford University Press, 2011); Kathleen Merikangas, Jian-ping He, Marcy Burstein, Sonja A. Swanson, and Shelli Avenevoli, "Lifetime Prevalence of Mental Disorders in US Adolescents: Results from the National Comorbidity Survey Replication—Adolescent Supplement (NCS-A)," *Journal of the American Academy of Child and Adolescent Psychiatry* 49, no. 10 (October 1, 2010): 980–89; H. Egger Bittner, A. Erkanli, Jane Costello, and D. Foley, "What Do Childhood Anxiety Disorders Predict?" *Journal of Child Psychology and Psychiatry* 48, no. 12 (October 2007): 1174–83.

2. E. Costello, S. Mustillo, A. Erkanli, G. Keeler, and A. Angold, "Prevalence and Development of Psychiatric Disorders in Childhood and Adolescence," *Archives of General Psychiatry* 60, no. 8 (August 2003): 837–44; Julia D. Buckner and Norman B. Schmidt, "Marijuana Effect Expectancies: Relations to Social Anxiety and Marijuana Use Problems," *Addictive Behaviors* 33, no. 11 (November 2008): 1477–83; P. C. Kendall, S. Safford, E. Flannery-Schroeder, and A. Webb, "Child Anxiety Treatment: Outcomes in Adolescence and Impact on Substance Use and Depression at 7.4-Year Follow-Up," *Journal of Consulting and Clinical Psychology* 72, no. 2 (April 2004): 276–87; L. J. Woodward and D.M. Fergusson, "Life Course Outcomes of Young People with Anxiety Disorders in Adolescence," *Journal of the American Academy of Child and Adolescent Psychiatry* 40, no. 9 (September 2001): 1086–93.

3. Kathryn A. Kerns, Shannon Siener, and Laura E. Brumariu, "Mother-Child Relationships, Family Context, and Child Characteristics as Predictors of Anxiety Symptoms in Middle Childhood," *Development and Psychopathology* 23, no. 2 (May 2011): 593–604.

4. Kathryn Degnan, Alisa Almas, and Nathan Fox, "Temperament and the Environment in the Etiology of Childhood Anxiety," *Journal of Child Psychology and Psychiatry* 51, no. 4 (April 2010): 497–517.

5. Allison M. Waters, Melanie J. Zimmer-Gembeck, and Lara J. Farrell, "The Relationships of Child and Parent Factors with Children Anxiety Symptoms: Parental Anxious Rearing as a Mediator," *Journal of Anxiety Disorders* 26, no. 7 (October 2012): 737–45.

6. Merel Kindt, "Malleability of Fear Memory: A Behavioral Neuroscience Perspective on the Etiology and Treatment of Anxiety Disorders," *Behavior Research and Therapy* 62 (September 2014): 24–36; Feng Lui, Chunyan Zhu, Yifeng Guo, Wenbin Li, and Meilling Wang, "Disrupted Cortical Hubs in Functional Brain Networks in Social Anxiety Disorder," *Clinical Neurophysiology* (November 27, 2014); Jeffrey Strawn, John Wegman, Keli Dominick, Max Swartz, and Anna Patinor, "Cortical Surface Anatomy in Pediatric Patients with Generalized Anxiety Disorder," *Journal of Anxiety Disorders* 28, no. 7 (October 2014): 717–23.

7. Shaozheng Qin, Christina Young, Tian Duan, Tianwen Chen, and Kaustubh Supekar, "Amygdala Subregional Structure and Intrinsic Functional Connectivity Predicts Individual Differences in Anxiety during Early Childhood," *Biological Psychiatry* 75, no. 11 (June 2014): 892–900.

8. Desmond J. Oathes, Brian Patenaude, Alan F. Schatzberg, and Amit Etkin, "Neurobiological Signatures of Anxiety and Depression in Resting-State Functional Magnetic Resonance Imaging," *Biological Psychiatry* 77, no. 4 (2015): 385–93.

9. Marta Andreatta, Evelyn Glotzbach-Schoon, Andreas Muhlberger, Stefan Schulz, and Julian Wiemer, "Initial and Sustained Brain Responses to Contextual Conditioned Anxiety in Humans," *Cortex* 63 (February 2015): 352–63; Jonathan Isper, Leesha Singh, and Dan Stein, "Meta-Analysis of Functional Brain Imaging in Specific Phobia," *Psychiatry and Clinical Neurosciences* 67, no. 5 (May 2013): 311–22; Melisa Carrasco, Christina Hong, Jenna Nienhuis, Shannon Harbin, and Kate Fitzgerald, "Increased Error Related Brain Activity in Youth with Obsessive Compulsive Disorder and Other Anxiety Disorders," *Neuroscience Letters* 541 (February 2013): 214–18.

10. Julia Zito, Daniel Safer, Susan dosReis, James Gardner, and Myde Boles, "Trends in the Prescribing of Psychotropic Medications to Preschoolers," *Journal of the American Medical Association* 283, no. 8 (February 2000): 1025–30; Thomas Delate, Alan Gelenberg, Valene Simmons, and Brenda Motheral, "Trends in the Use of Antidepressants in a National Sample of Commercially Insured Pediatric Patients, 1998–2002," *Psychiatric Services* 55 (2004): 387–91.

11. Wendy Silverman, A. Pina, and Chockalivgam Viswesvaran, "Evidence-based Psychosocial Treatments for Phobic and Anxiety Disorders in Children and Adolescents," *Journal of Clinical Child and Adolescent Psychology* 37, no. 1 (2008): 105–30; D. Chambless and S. Hollon, "Defining Empirically Supported Therapies," *Journal of Consulting and Clinical Psychology* 66, no. 1 (February 1998): 7–18; S. Hollon and A. Beck, "Cognitive and Cognitive Behavioral Therapies," in *Bergin and Garfield's Handbook of Psychotherapy and Behavioral Change*, 6th ed., ed. M. J. Lambert, 393–442 (New York: Wiley, 2013); T. Ollendick and N. King, "Evidence-based Treatments for Children and Adolescents: Issues and Commentary," in *Child and*

Adolescent Therapy: Cognitive Behavioral Procedures, 4th ed., ed. P. C. Kendall, 499–520 (New York: Guilford Press, 2011).

12. Dina Hirshfeld-Becker, Jamie Micco, Heather Mazursky, L. Bruett, and A. Henin, "Applying Cognitive-Behavioral Therapy for Anxiety to the Younger Child," *Child and Adolescent Clinics of North America* 20, no. 2 (April 2011): 349–68.

13. Paula Barrett, Amanda Duffy, Mark Dadds, and Ronald Rapee, "Cognitive Behavioral Treatment of Anxiety Disorders in Children: Long Term Follow Up," *Journal of Consulting and Clinical Psychology* 69, no. 1 (February 2001): 135–41; Courtney Benjamin, Julie Harrison, Cara Settipani, Douglas Brodman, and Philip Kendall, "Anxiety and Related Outcomes in Young Adults 7–19 Years after Receiving Treatment for Child Anxiety," *Journal of Consulting and Clinical Psychology* 81, no. 5 (2013): 865–76; P. C. Kendall et al., "Child Anxiety Treatment"; Laura Seligman and Thomas Ollendick, "Cognitive Behavioral Treatment for Anxiety Disorders in Youth," *Child and Adolescent Psychiatric Clinics of North America* 20, no. 2 (April 2012): 217–38.

14. K. Brendel and B. Maynard, "Child-Parent Interventions for Childhood Anxiety," *Research on Social Work Practice* 24, no. 3 (2014): 287–95; Jennifer Podell and Phillip Kendall, "Mothers and Fathers in Family Cognitive Behavioral Therapy for Anxious Youth," *Journal of Child and Family Studies* 20, no. 2 (2011): 182–95; John Piacentini, Lyndey Bergman, Susanna Chang, Audra Langley, and Tara Peris, "Controlled Comparison of Family Cognitive Behavioral Therapy and Psychoeducation: Relaxation Training for Child Obsessive Compulsive Disorder," *Journal of the Academy of Child and Adolescent Psychiatry* 50, no. 11 (2011): 1149–61; Barbara Esbiorn, Michael Somhovd, Sara Nielsen, Nicole Normann, and Ingrid Leth, "Parental Changes after Involvement in Their Anxious Child's Cognitive Behavioral Treatment," *Journal of Anxiety Disorders* 28, no. 7 (October 2014): 664–70; Allison Smith, Ellen Flannery-Schroeder, Kathleen Gorman, and Nathan Cook, "Parent Cognitive Behavioral Intervention for the Treatment of Childhood Anxiety Disorders: A Pilot Study," *Behavior Research and Therapy* 61 (October 2014): 156–61; Kirsten Thirlwall, Peter Cooper, Jessica Karalus, Merryn Voysey, and Lucy Willetts, "Treatment of Child Anxiety Disorders via Guided Parent-Delivered Cognitive-Behavioral Therapy: Randomised Controlled Trial," *British Journal of Psychiatry* 203, no. 6 (December 2013): 436–44.

15. Patricia Porto, Leticia Oliveira, Jair Mari, Elaine Volchan, and Ivan Figueira, "Does Cognitive Behavioral Therapy Change the Brain? A Systematic Review of Neuroimaging in Anxiety Disorders," *Journal of Neuropsychiatry and Clinical Neurosciences* 21, no. 2 (2009): 114–25; Vincent Paquette, Johanne Levesque, Boualem Mensour, Jean-Maxime Leroux, and Gilles Beaudoin, "'Change the Mind and You Change the Brain': Effects of Cognitive-Behavioral Therapy on the Neural Correlates of Spider Phobia," *Neuroimage* 18, no. 2 (February 2003): 401–9; Andrea Reinecke, Kai Thilo, Nicola Filippini, Alison Croft, and Catherine Harmer, "Predicting Rapid Response to Cognitive-Behavioral Treatment for Panic Disorder: The Role of Hippocampus, Insula, and Dorsolateral Prefrontal Cortex," *Behavior*

Research and Therapy 62 (November 2014): 120–28; Ulrike Leuken, Benjamin Straube, Carten Konrad, Hans Wittchen, and Andreas Strohle, "Neural Substrates of Treatment Response to Cognitive-Behavioral Therapy in Panic Disorder with Agoraphobia," *American Journal of Psychiatry* 170, no. 11 (November 2013): 1345–55; Phillipe Golden, Mifal Ziv, Hooria Jazaieri, Justin Weeks, and Richard Heimberg, "Impact of Cognitive-Behavioral Therapy for Social Anxiety Disorder on the Neural Bases of Emotional Reactivity to and Regulation of Social Evaluation," *Behavior Research and Therapy* 62 (November 2014): 97–106; V. Miskovic, D. Moscovitch, D. Santesso, R. McCabe, and M. Antony, "Changes in EEG Cross-Frequency Coupling during Cognitive Behavioral Therapy for Social Anxiety Disorder," *Psychological Science* 22, no. 4 (April 2011): 507–16; J. Strawn, A. Wehry, M. DelBello, M. Rynn, and S. Strakowski, "Establishing the Neurobiological Basis of Treatment in Children and Adolescents with Generalized Anxiety Disorder," *Depression and Anxiety* 29, no. 4 (April 2012): 328–39.

16. Eli Lebowitz, Lyndsey Scharfstein, and Johanna Jones, "Comparing Family Accommodation in Pediatric Obsessive-Compulsive Disorder, Anxiety Disorders, and Nonanxious Children," *Depression and Anxiety* 31, no. 12 (December 2014): 1018–25; Johanna Thompson-Hollands, Caroline Kerns, Donna Pincus, and Jonathan Comer, "Parental Accommodation of Child Anxiety and Related Symptoms: Range, Impact, and Correlates," *Journal of Anxiety Disorders* 28, no. 8 (December 2014): 765–73; C. Wei and P. Kendall, "Child Perceived Parenting Behavior: Childhood Anxiety and Related Symptoms," *Child and Family Behavior Therapy* 36, no. 1 (January 2014): 1–18.

17. Hirshfeld-Becker et al., "Applying Cognitive-Behavioral Therapy."

18. Martina Gere, Marianne Villabo, Sven Torgersen, and Phillip Kendall, "Overprotective Parenting and Child Anxiety: The Role of Co-occurring Child Behavior Problems," *Journal of Anxiety Disorders* 26, no. 6 (August 2012): 642–49.

19. J. Silk, L. Sheeber, P. Tan, C. Ladouceur, and E. Forbes, "You Can Do It!' The Role of Parental Encouragement of Bravery in Child Anxiety Treatment," *Journal of Anxiety Disorders* 27, no. 5 (June 2013): 439–46.

Index

abuse of benzodiazepines, 225

accommodation, educational, 228–29

accommodation, parental: avoidance and, 10–11; problems with, 13–14; separation anxiety, 92, 111; specific phobias, 164–66

ADHD (attention deficit hyperactivity disorder): *DSM-5* diagnostic criteria for, 63–65; GAD and, 60–61

advocates for working with school system, 230

agreeing on challenges to work on, 22–23; GAD, 43–44, 55–56; OCD, 129–31, 139–40; PTSD, 178–79, 191–92; selective mutism, 72–73; separation anxiety, 99–100, 113; social anxiety, 84–85; specific phobias, 157–58, 169

alcohol and drug addictions: abuse of benzodiazepines, 225; anxiety and, 5; faith in pills and, 224; GAD and, 50–52; social anxiety and, 82

amygdala, 6

anger: of child, over anxiety problems, 40, 96, 223; oppositional behavior and anxiety, 84; of parent, at child's anxiety, 10, 92; as resistance and denial, 79–80; at therapist, 97

anterior cingulate cortex, 6

anxiety disorders, 4–5; ADHD and, 60–61; biological underpinnings of, 5–8, 11; irrationality of anxiety, 90; prevalence of, 1; resistance and, 79–80, 172–73; social isolation and, 31, 82; tantrums and, 8, 36, 92. *See also* physical symptoms; talking back to anxiety; targeting anxious thoughts and behaviors; *specific disorders*

Asperger syndrome and bug phobia, 161–66

attention deficit hyperactivity disorder (ADHD): *DSM-5* diagnostic criteria for, 63–65; GAD and, 60–61

autism spectrum disorders: communication difficulties and, 77; selective mutism and, 67

avoidance: as common reaction, 19; complaints of pain and, 231; as defense against anxiety, 13, 20, 34; enabling of, 172; parental accommodation and, 10–11; social anxiety and, 81; targeting, 83

bathroom at school, using, 76

behavioral part of CBT, 13

behaviors: normalizing, 31, 41, 71, 85, 192; oppositional, and anxiety, 84, 96. *See also* rating anxious behaviors; targeting anxious thoughts and behaviors; targeting behaviors

benzodiazepines, 225

biological underpinnings of anxiety, 5–8

brain: experience as changing, 13; "fear circuitry" of, 5–7; plasticity of, 9–10

bugs, fear of, 161–66

bullying, 226–27

calendar format for charting progress, 26–27, 28–29

calm-down list: fear of vomiting, 24; GAD, 45–46; separation anxiety, 114–15

campus, rape on, 183–85, 190, 195

case studies, 2; fear of vomiting, 17–20; GAD, 35–40, 49–53; hair pulling, 203–12; OCD, 122–25, 135–37; PTSD,

neuropsychological evaluation, 60–61, 229–30

normalizing behavior, 31, 41, 71, 85, 192

Note and Chart Progress Made. *See* progress, noting and charting of

obsessions: anxiety-driven movements, 215–17; hair pulling, 209

obsessive compulsive disorder (OCD), 120–21; and agreeing on challenges to work on, 129–31, 139–40; case studies of, 122–25, 135–37; genetic component of, 121; and incentives to motivate, 133, 143–44; and noting and charting progress, 132, 142–43; and rating anxious behavior, 128, 138–39; and reinforcing progress and increasing challenges, 133–34, 144–45; and strategies to practice, 131–32, 140–42; and targeting anxious thoughts and behaviors, 126–27, 137–38; tics and, 216–17

Offer Incentives to Motivate. *See* incentives to motivate

oppositional behavior, 84, 96

overmedication, 223–24

overprotective parenting, 11–12

PANDAS (pediatric autoimmune neuropsychological disorder associated with strep), 121, 132, 133

panic attacks, 7, 192

parenting, 10–12, 232

parents, 14; as advocates, 230; anxious, 11; involvement of, in treatment, 9, 12–13; as overprotective, 11–12; support for, 232–35. *See also* accommodation, parental; team approach

pediatric autoimmune neuropsychological disorder associated with strep (PANDAS), 121, 132, 133

pediatricians: antianxiety medication and, 224; medical evaluations and, 230

perceptions of surroundings, 7

perfectionism and learning, 33–34, 53

phobias. *See* fear; selective mutism; specific phobias

physical symptoms: of anxiety, 6; of GAD, 34–35, 36–37; headaches, 219, 223; phobic reactions, 149; of separation anxiety, 91–92, 104, 109; stomach problems, 218–19, 230. *See also* sleep problems

pica, 208

picky eating, 217–18

plasticity of brain, 9–10

post-traumatic stress disorder (PTSD), 175; and agreeing on challenges to work on, 178–79, 191–92; case studies of, 176, 183–85; in children six years and younger, 198–201; *DSM-5* diagnostic criteria for, 195–98; and incentives to motivate, 180, 193; and noting and charting progress, 180, 193; and rating anxious behaviors, 177, 191; and reinforcing progress and increasing challenges, 180–82, 194; and strategies to practice, 179–80, 192; and targeting anxious thoughts and behaviors, 177, 186–91

practicing CBT strategies, 12. *See also* strategies to practice

prevalence of anxiety disorders, 1

progress, noting and charting of, 26–27, 28–29; GAD, 46, 58; OCD, 132, 142–43; PTSD, 180, 193; selective mutism, 74; separation anxiety, 101–2, 115; social anxiety, 86; specific phobias, 159, 170

progress, reinforcing, 30–31; and GAD, 47–49, 59–60; and OCD, 133–34, 144–45; and PTSD, 180–82, 194; and separation anxiety, 102–3, 116–17; and specific phobias, 160–61, 171–72

protecting child from anxiety, 25. *See also* accommodation, parental

Prozac, 104–5, 117, 204